Smart Sanitation Solutions

Examples of innovative, low-cost technologies for toilets, collection, transportation, treatment and use of sanitation products

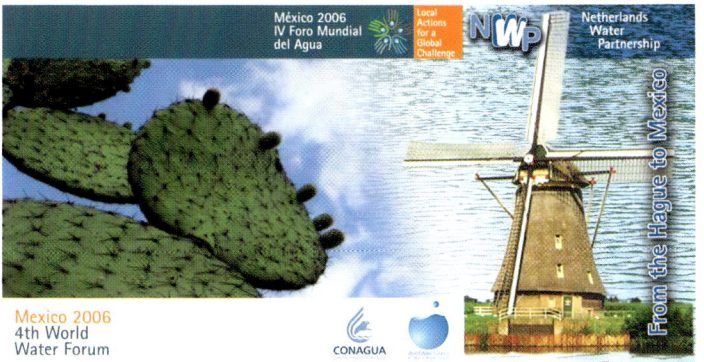

The first edition of this booklet was drafted as a contribution to the Fourth World Water Forum in Mexico in March 2006 in a collaboration between the Netherlands Water Partnership, WASTE, PRACTICA, IRC and SIMAVI. Partners for Water financially supported this edition.

Collaboration

Based on the success of the series Smart Water Solutions, and the increased interest in appropriate sanitation solutions, this edition shares information on sanitation technologies. It is designed as a source of inspiration, rather than a 'how to' manual.

This publication is a collaborative effort by five organisations:

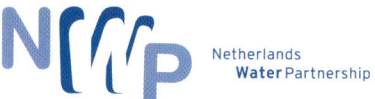

NWP, the Netherlands Water Partnership, is an independent organisation formed by government bodies, NGOs, knowledge institutes, and businesses involved in the water sector.
The main aim of the NWP is to harmonise initiatives of the Dutch water sector and to promote Dutch water expertise worldwide. www.nwp.nl

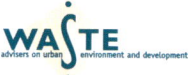

WASTE advisers on urban environment and development works towards sustainable improvement in the living conditions of the urban poor and in the urban environment. Long-term, multi-country programmes and projects have a focus on bottom-up development in relation to recycling, solid waste management, ecological sanitation, and knowledge sharing. www.waste.n

PRACTICA

The **PRACTICA Foundation** facilitates the exchange of knowledge on, and the development of, innovative and low-cost water technologies.
www.practicafoundation.nl

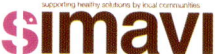

Simavi supports health and healthcare initiatives in developing countries with a focus on water and sanitation activities. www.simavi.org

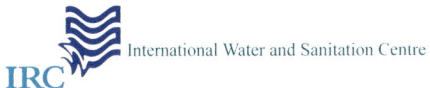

IRC International Water and Sanitation Centre provides news, publishing, documentation and portal services, helping partners with capacity building for pro-poor sustainable water supply, sanitation, and hygiene in developing countries. www.irc.nl

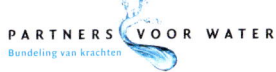

Publication of this booklet has been funded by **Partners for Water**, a programme that aims to strengthen the international position of the Dutch water sector by uniting forces (companies, departments, NGOs and knowledge institutes). Partners for Water is overseen by the Dutch Agency for International Business and Cooperation (EVD) in collaboration with the Netherlands Water Partnership (NWP).
More information: www.partnersforwater.nl

Also Available in this series:
- Smart Water Solutions (ISBN 978 94 6022 005 0) Also available in Portuguese, French and Spanish
- Smart Water Harvesting Solutions (ISBN 978 94 6022 004 3) Also available in Portuguese en French
- Smart Finance Solutions (ISBN 978 94 6022 010 4)

© 2009 by NWP, second edition
All rights reserved. Reproduction permitted for non-commercial use.
© 2009 KIT Publishers, Amsterdam, The Netherlands
Email: publishers@kit.nl
Website: www.kit.nl/publishers

Text:	WASTE
Editing:	IRC/Peter McIntyre
Graphic design:	Aforma Drukkerij, Apeldoorn
Printing:	High Trade, Zwolle
Financial support:	Partners for Water
Cover photo:	WaterAid, Caroline Penn

ISBN 978 94 6022 002 9

Table of contents

Foreword — 5
The need for sanitation — 6
Factors influencing pathogen die-off — 8
The challenges of sanitation coverage — 9
What makes sanitation technologies smart? — 10
The elements of sanitation technologies — 11
Figures on the characteristics of excreta — 14

Sanitation techniques — 15
    An all in one system; *the ArborLoo* — 17

Toilets
    Dry toilets — 19
    Dry urine diversion toilets — 21
    Pour flush slabs — 23
    Waterless urinals — 25

Collection
    Fossa Alterna — 27
    Oil drums and containers — 29
    Vaults and chambers — 31

Transportation
    Cartage system — 33
    MAPET and Vacutug system — 35
    Settled sewerage (small diameter) — 37

Treatment
    Co-composting — 39
    Dehydration — 41
    Planted soil filter — 43
    Anaerobic digestion — 45

Using sanitation products
    Intermezzo "The need to recover phosphorous from excreta" — 47
    Compost as soil conditioner — 49
    Human urine as fertiliser — 51
    Biogas as source of energy — 53

Case study 1: Urine diversion in the Philippines — 55
Case study 2: Fixed-dome biogas systems in Nepal — 61
Some terminology used in this booklet — 67
Call for information — 68

Foreword

Scepticism about achieving essential development goals and fighting poverty is fading away. Since the Millennium Development Summit in 2000, when 189 heads of state declared their full commitment to achieving the eight Millennium Development Goals (MDGs), the world has had an unprecedented opportunity to improve the living conditions of billions of people in rural and urban areas. MDG 7 is particularly relevant to this booklet. Target 10 of that goal is to halve the proportion of people without sustainable access to safe drinking water and improved sanitation by 2015. The Netherlands is ready to take concrete steps in this field and that is why I pledged in 2005 to contribute towards providing access to safe drinking water and sanitation for at least fifty million people by 2015.

The time for lengthy discussions is over. Now it is time for action. Political will, increased resources, affordable technologies and new partnerships are in place to increase access to safe drinking water and sanitation. We must realise, however, that most sanitation facilities used by households or operated by small-scale enterprises were built without external support. This shows there are alternatives to the large centralised conventional systems. More importantly, small-scale solutions have proven to be cost effective. Implemented in large numbers, they can boost health, improve agricultural production and generate local business all at the same time. That is why large-scale dissemination of these technologies is crucial. Smart technologies like this help us to tackle poverty immediately. Capacity building in both software and hardware is equally important to success – not only for users and institutions, but also for small and medium-sized enterprises.

This booklet on sanitation, like its counterpart Smart Water Solutions, gives examples of household and community-based sanitation solutions that have proven effective and affordable. It illustrates a range of innovative sanitation technologies that have already helped thousands of poor families to improve their lives. The technologies described are a source of inspiration.

Finally, I would like to express my hope that sharing this information will bring "Sanitation for All" closer to reality!

Agnes van Ardenne
Minister for Development Cooperation
The Netherlands

The need for sanitation

In 2004, the World Health Organization estimated that about 1.8 million people die every year from diarrhoeal diseases (including cholera). About 90% of these deaths are of children under 5 years of age.
Sanitation conditions at school heavily influence school attendance, especially by girls. Lack of facilities or unhygienic conditions not only prevent children participating in school, they also negatively affect their concentration and ability to learn. For example, in Madagascar alone, 3.5 million schooldays are lost each year due to ill-health, related to poor sanitation. Many adolescent girls drop out of school because of appalling and unsafe toilet conditions.

World Health Organization, Water, Sanitation and Hygiene Links to Health Facts and figures, 2004
- 88% of diarrhoeal disease is attributed to unsafe water supply, inadequate sanitation and hygiene.
- Improved water supply reduces diarrhoea by between 6% and 25%.
- Improved sanitation reduces diarrhoea by 32%.

Sanitation, along with clean water and food security, is a primary driver for improving public health. It reduces people's exposure to disease by providing a clean living environment. It is a crucial element in breaking the cycle of infection-disease-recovery-infection, resulting from unsafe disposal of human waste containing pathogens. Behavioural and technical measures are both required to create a hygienic environment. Critical measures include hand washing before cooking, and boiling or chlorinating drinking water.

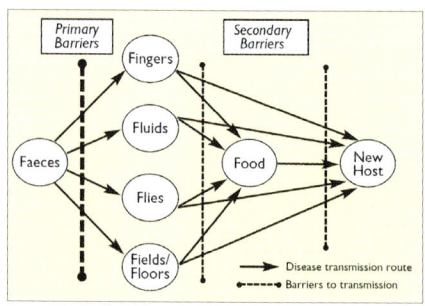

Disease transmission and control

(Source: Water and Sanitation Collaborative Council and World Health Organization, Sanitation and Hygiene Promotion, Programming Guidance, 2005)

"Independent of the type of toilets provided, interventions including the whole water and sanitation system are important to improve the health situation."
(Schönning, Stenström, 2004. For more information visit the Swedish Institute for Disease Control www.smi.ki.se)

"A review study on the impact of hand washing with soap, concerning the risk of diarrhoeal diseases showed that washing hands with soap could reduce the risk of diarrhoeal diseases by 42 to 47%."
(Fewtrell & Colford, 2004)

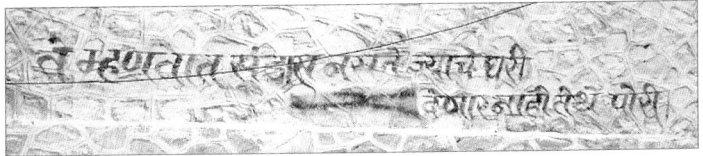

"Daughters from our village do not marry into villages where open defecation is practiced."
(Wall writings in Matathi language in Borban village of Ahmednagar district in Maharashtra state in India)
(Source: IDS Working Paper 184, Subsidy or Self-Respect? Participatory Total Community Sanitation in Bangladesh, Kamal Kar, 2003)

There is a wide range of different diseases and transmission pathways, which means that improvements depend on a large number of people changing a wide range of behaviours and conditions. In practice, people are more motivated by social ambition than by health arguments. Improving the family's status is an important motivation in adopting better hygiene practices and being willing to pay for sanitation. Other incentives are privacy, safety and convenience, and to reduce health care costs.

"Where local builders benefit directly from projects they become effective champions for sanitation improvement, and help build local demand!"
(Kathy Eales and Richard Holden, The Mvula Trust)

Potential champions for improving sanitation can be found in every community, as can people with the necessary building and organisational skills. Family members and the local private sector are often the primary designers and providers of sanitation services. These activities contribute to the improvement of the livelihoods in a community.
Sanitary officials and public heath workers play an important role in facilitating private entrepreneurs and the creating awareness about the importance of proper hygiene and sanitation.

Factors influencing pathogen die-off

Pathogens die off after excretion, as environmental conditions outside the human host are generally not favourable to their survival. Environmental factors that contribute to the die-off of pathogens are listed in the table below.[1]

Factor	Description
Nutrients	Pathogens living in the gut are not always capable of competing with other organisms outside the body for scarce nutrients.
Temperature	Most microorganisms survive at low temperatures (<5 °C) and rapidly die off at high temperatures (>40-50 °C) during composting and/or dehydration.
pH	Many microorganisms are adapted to a neutral pH (7). Increasing acidic or alkaline conditions through adding ash or lime will have an inactivating effect.
Dryness	Moist conditions favour the survival of microorganism. Dry conditions decrease the number of pathogens.
Solar radiation / UV light	The survival time of pathogens will be shorter when they are exposed to sunlight (when excreta are applied to the soil).
Presence of other organisms	Organisms may affect each other by predation, release of substances or competition as happens when waste water is treated in soil filters or excreta is applied in agriculture.
Oxygen	Microbiological activity is dependent on oxygen. Most pathogens are anaerobic and are likely to be out-competed by other organisms in an aerobic environment. For this reason, application of excreta to soil and exposure to ventilation contributes to die-off.
Time	All the above conditions only become relevant in relation to time. In other words, the more time pathogens are exposed to these conditions, the less chance they have of surviving.

[1] 2004-1, Guidelines on the Safe Use of Urine and Faeces in Ecological sanitation Systems, Schönning and Stenström

The challenges of sanitation coverage

"Water and Sanitation is one of the primary drivers of public health. I often refer to it as "Health 101", which means that once we can secure access to clean water and to adequate sanitation facilities for all people, irrespective of the difference in their living conditions, a huge battle against all kinds of diseases will be won."
Dr LEE Jong-wook, Director-General, World Health Organization, 2004.

It is a major challenge to "halve by 2015 the proportion of people without sustainable access to safe drinking water and basic sanitation" (MDG 7, Target 10). Only through a considerable increase in the construction and improvement of sanitation facilities within the next ten years, can the sanitation target be achieved.

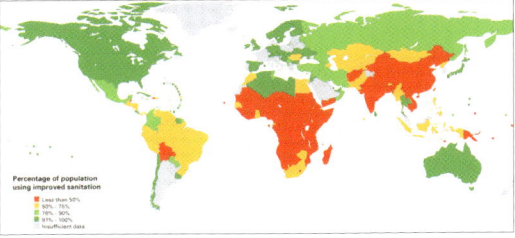

Progress in sanitation coverage 1990 - 2002 (Unicef and WHO).

The main challenges in reaching the MDG sanitation target are:
- Senior officials and politicians must convince themselves about the importance of sanitation for public health, economic development and the dignity of people;
- To improve awareness and knowledge among decision makers about the vital link between sanitation and health, and the relation between sanitation and economic development;
- Sanitation improvement has to be based on cultural preferences, and take account of traditional behaviours and practices;
- Intelligent use has to be made of (always scarce) financial resources through the involvement of entrepreneurs and other key stakeholders;
- Informed demand for improved sanitation must be stimulated, offering people information about appropriate (smart) technologies and services.

Sanitation facilities are only sustainable when people make their own choices and own contribution towards obtaining and maintaining them. People have to experience the toilet as an improvement in their daily life. Sanitation systems have to be embedded in the local institutional, financial-economic, social-cultural, legal-political, and environmental context.

What makes sanitation technologies *smart*?

Besides constituting an effective disease barrier, *smart* sanitation solutions prevent environmental pollution and optimise the use of resource in terms of nutrients, water and energy. Sanitation must meet the needs of the user, must be simple to use, to maintain and repair, be possible to replicate and be affordable.

A sanitation technology is *'smart'* when adapted to local conditions and adaptable to changing environment.
The same technology may be smart in a Mexican city but not be adequate when applied in an Indian slum.

To develop a *smart* sanitation solution in a local context, the following guidelines are crucial:
- Involving families and the private sector in design and planning (developing ownership);
- Responding to actual needs (demand responsive);
- Building on existing practice, experience and infrastructure (don't re-invent the wheel);
- Taking account of values, attitudes and behaviour of the users (culturally sensitive);
- Making choices based on affordability and willingness to pay;
- Considering existing institutional settings (develop institutional support).

Further information about a variety of approaches and methodologies that have been developed to tackle the above issues can be found through ITDG, IRC, GHK Research & Training, WASTE and others.

ITDG	www.itdg.org
IRC	www.irc.nl
GHK Research & Training	www.ghkint.com
WASTE	www.waste.nl

The elements of sanitation technologies

"I prefer to talk about 'sanitation' rather than 'toilets'. A flush toilet is basically a machine for mixing human urine, faeces and water. Sanitation, on the other hand, is a system."
Uno Winblad

A sanitation system does not solely refer to toilets. Toilets are only one element in an entire sanitation system.
Other elements such as collection, transport, treatment, and use of excreta are all together vital for sustainable sanitation.

Dividing the sanitation system into five elements creates considerable room for flexibility in design and choice in developing an appropriate solution adapted to local conditions. A wide range of practices exists for each element. However, flexibility of choice is limited because some combinations do not work. For example, a dry toilet can not be combined with a sewer network.

Toilets
A toilet is a primary barrier between people and the pathogens present in faeces, because it contains the collection of excreta in a designated and controlled location. In addition to the toilet itself, the facility should include the means for hand-washing and provide privacy, safety and comfort to the user. These features are all important for the functioning of the entire sanitation system. Toilet options are the main focus of this booklet.

Further information on hand washing and superstructures can be found through:
IRC	www.irc.nl
WEDC	www.wedc.lboro.ac.uk
WHO	www.who.int
WSSCC	www.wsscc.org
CSIR	www.csir.co.za

Toilet designs are *smart* when hygienic safety is guaranteed, and excreta can be dealt with in a socio-culturally acceptable way. Toilets must be seen by the relevant population as safe and attractive to use, while construction and maintenance costs have to be affordable.

Collection
A collection facility aims to prevent the uncontrolled dispersal of material containing pathogens. The collection facility, which often needs ventilation, safely contains human excreta awaiting transportation. Some collection facilities include pre-treatment of excreta. In addition, to these important functions, a smart collection facility makes efficient use of limited space and can function effectively over a long period.

Transportation
A transportation system is crucial when excreta can't be treated, deposited or used onsite. Good organisation and management of transportation systems will determine the sustainability and continuity of the entire sanitation system.

Transportation systems can be divided into infrastructure base systems, such as sewer networks, or logistic management using regular transportation means such as trucks, vacuum tankers, carts, and tricycles. Sewer networks require sufficient water to transport excreta effectively.

Whether sewerage (i.e. the drainage system in which sewage is transported) is appropriate heavily depends on soil conditions, the availability of sufficient amounts of water for flushing (now and in the future), and the availability of financial and institutional capacity.

Factors that influence the design and applicability of the transport system include the amount of waste generated, housing density, street access, haul distance, road conditions, road gradient, traffic type, and the cost of labour and fuel. A house-to-house collector may transport material directly to its destination. However, transfer becomes necessary when distances increase and direct transport is no longer economically feasible or when the destination can only be reached with a different means of transport.

Treatment
Treatment aims at reducing the level of pathogens in excreta with a final aim of achieving total die-off, to prevent infection of people and pollution of the environment.

A smart designer of a treatment system also considers the recovery of resources, notably nutrients, present in excreta. Appropriate treatment systems are *smart* when they are designed based on the required characteristics of the end-product (for economic use). This 'reversed sanitation design' approach will also have consequences for the previous elements. For example, keeping excreta separate from grey water and storm water, or keeping urine and faeces separate provides options for more efficient recovery of resources.

Treatment facilities are either located on-site, or off-site, depending on land availability and reuse potential of excreta and grey water. If reuse of treated excreta is appropriate at the household level, on-site treatment is preferred.

To avoid health risks, handling of excreta must be limited and controlled. In most circumstances, on-site treatments meet these concerns.

Two treatment stages

Primary treatment	Reducing volumes, weight and pathogens in order to facilitate safe storage, transportation and further (secondary) treatment.
Secondary treatment	Controlled treatment to reduce pathogens to acceptable limits.

Using sanitation products

Sanitation not only contributes to public health and environmental protection. *Smart* sanitation can also contribute to global food security. The 'market' consists mainly of farmers who are therefore major stakeholders in the design of this element.

Reuse, recycling, and recovery all refer in some way to the extraction and/or utilisation of materials and energy from excreta or wastewater. The nutrients in excreta have a high fertilising value, and can partly replace the demand for artificial fertiliser. Excreta can improve soil conditions and generate biogas. Biogas can be used in households for cooking and heating.

If excreta and/or wastewater cannot be used or processed in some way, it needs to be disposed of. Ways must be found to dispose of excreta while taking into account the serious threat to public health and the environment posed by improper handling. Uncontrolled disposal of excreta in soil or water can also overload organic compounds and nutrients in the environment, resulting in the loss of plant and animal life.

Figures on the characteristics of excreta

Characteristics	Urine	Faeces
Volume* (WHO, 1992)		
High-protein diet, temperate climate	440 l/cap/y	44 kg/cap/y
Vegetarian diet, tropical climate	370 l/cap/y	146 kg/cap/y
Pathogen content	Usually sterile	High
Nutrient content (SEPA, 1995 and Wolfgast, 1993)		
Nitrogen (N) phosphorous (P) and potassium (K)		
% N of total excreted amount	70% - 88%	12% - 30%
% P of total excreted amount	25% - 67%	33% - 75%
% K of total excreted amount	71%	29%
Relative organic content	Low	High

*l/cap/y – litre per capita per year (the amount excreted in one year, by one person

Volume of excreta (urine and faeces)
The volume of faeces and urine varies from region to region and depends on climate, the age of a person, their water consumption, diet, and occupation.
Diet influences the volume of faeces according to the digestibility of the food. The amount of urine also depends on temperature and humidity.

Pathogen content
Urine leaving the human body usually contains no pathogens. On the other hand, faeces contain microorganisms, including pathogens among which are bacteria, viruses, parasitic protozoa, and helminths.

Nutrient content
The nutrient content of excreta varies according to the differences in diet (digestibility of the food). However, in general the nutrient content of urine is much higher than the nutrient content of faeces.

Other substances to think of
Excreta contains little heavy metal and few other contaminating substances (e.g. pesticide residues). The amount depends on the amounts present in consumed products. Hormones and residuals of medicines (pharmaceuticals) are excreted with urine. These are degraded in the ground by soil microbes and vegetation.

Sanitation techniques

This booklet illustrates a selection of *smart* sanitation technologies, although it does not set out to be comprehensive or to be a manual. However, the booklet does hope to become a source of inspiration for those who are trying to improve sanitation conditions.

The techniques described in this booklet, according to the elements making up entire sanitation systems:

Toilets	Collection	Transportation	Treatment	Use of products
	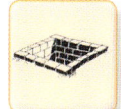		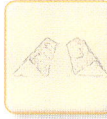	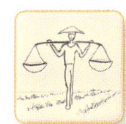
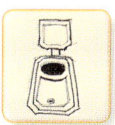	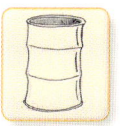	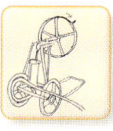	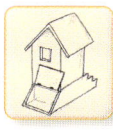	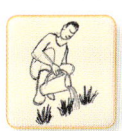
	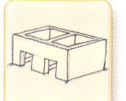	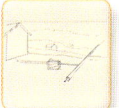	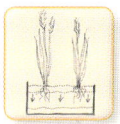	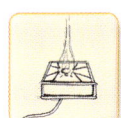
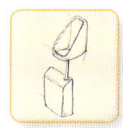			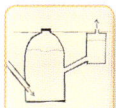	

Example:

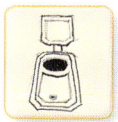 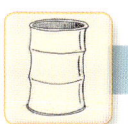 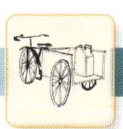  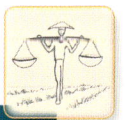

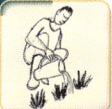

Toilets

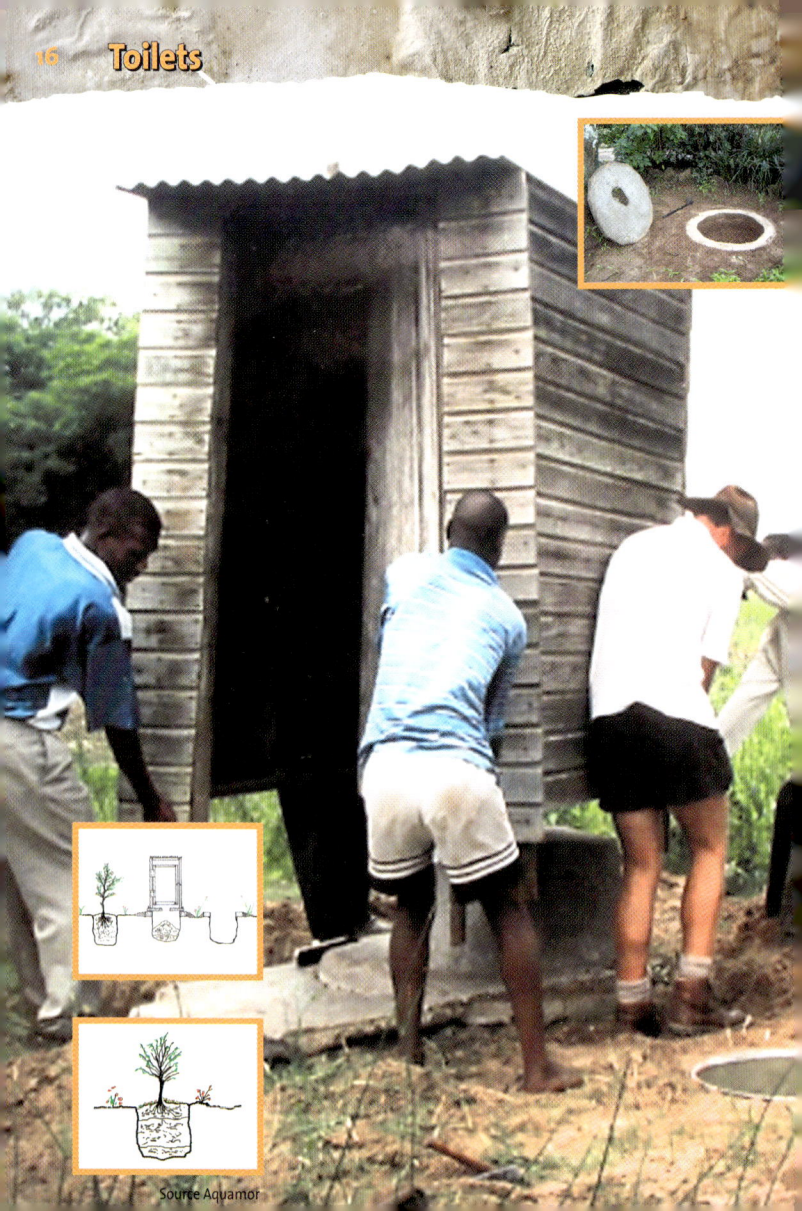

Source Aquamor

An all in one system; the *ArborLoo*

ArborLoo systems consist of a dry toilet, placed above a shallow pit about 1 metre deep. The shallow pit is usually dug by hand on which an elevated ring beam and slab are placed. Excreta is deposited into the pit and covered with soil after each use. In the pit, excreta is composted. This process can be improved by adding wood ash and leaves. When the pit is nearly full (about 6-9 months for one family), the toilet and superstructure are removed and the pit is filled with additional soil. The toilet and superstructure are transferred to a new pit and the process is repeated. A tree is planted on top of the filled pit. Because the system includes all the elements of a sanitation system – a toilet, a collection pit, a composting process, and a composted site to grow a tree – the *ArborLoo* system can be seen as an all-in-one-system.

Applying conditions

- *ArborLoos* can be applied in very scattered communities as well as in urban and peri-urban areas. If space is limited, trees such as pawpaws that provide fruit and shade can be planted. Alternatively, a full pit can be left to compost for a year, and the compost can be dug out.
- All toilets should be built on slightly raised ground to avoid surface flooding; the pits should be shallow where water tables are high.
- The conversion of excreta into humus will not take place if the pit is flooded with water. Therefore, good pit drainage is necessary. In case wet anal cleaning is preferred above wiping, a special washing area should be provided.
- In areas with an unstable soil, the ring beam elevating the slab is placed a little deeper. In very loose collapsing sandy soil, the pit must be lined. If it is intended to excavate the compost rather than planting a tree, then two pits could be dug, to be used alternately.
- Alternatively, since pit compost is easier to dig out than parent soil, this system is often used with two alternate pits to make compost that is dug out after a year.

Costs:	Toilet slab	US$ 2 (Malawi, Zimbabwe).
	ArborLoo (per 100 units)	US$ 5 – 15 (Zimbabwe).

Advantages:	**Disadvantages:**
Minimal contact with faeces.	Only where is sufficient space.
Easy to construct.	Toilet cleaning of the toilet must be done with small amounts of water.
No handling of fresh excreta.	Water used for anal cleaning should be collected separate.

Information:	General	www.wsp.org
		www.wateraid.org.uk
	Zimbabwe	http://aquamor.tripod.com

Moving an *ArborLoo* superstructure in Maputoland (photo Aquamor).
Insert: A hole is dug down within the ring beam (photo Aquamor).

Toilets

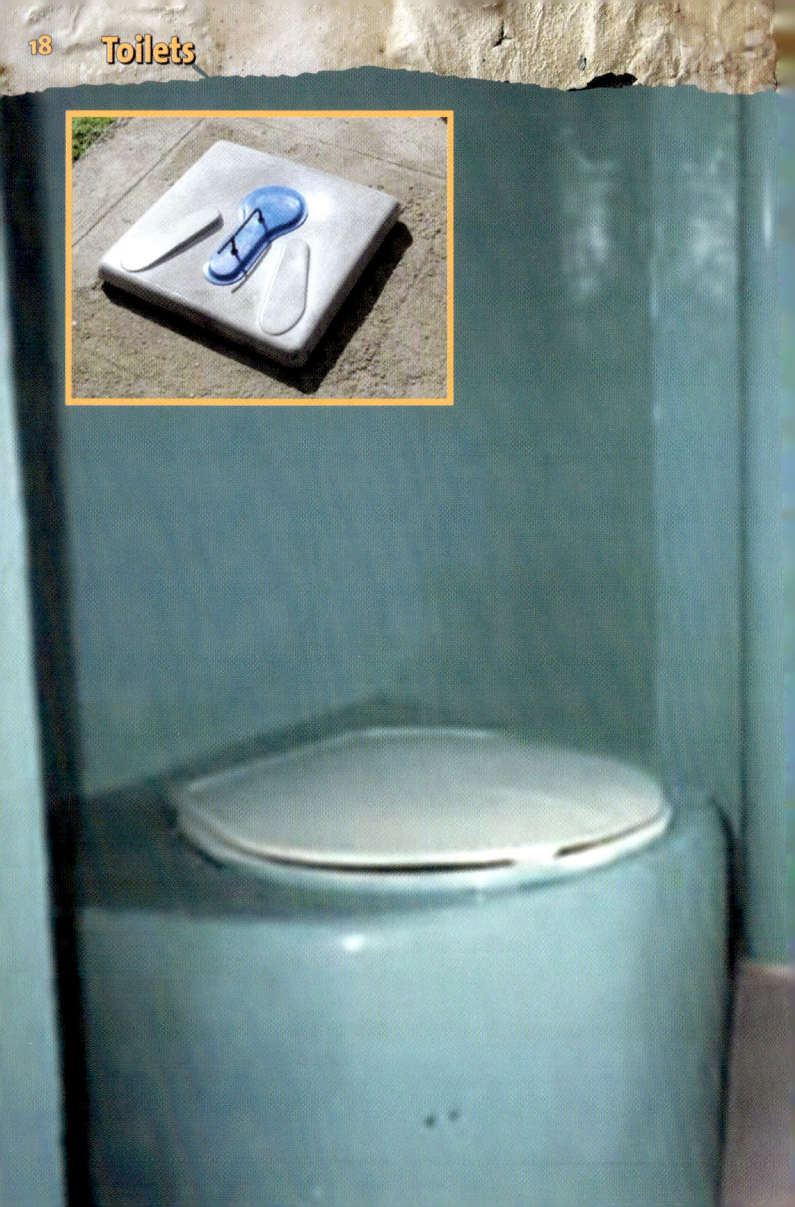

Dry toilets

A dry toilet differs from a flush toilet (Water Closet) in that it does not need water. Excreta are collected directly beneath the seat in a shallow pit, container, chamber, etc. The system should not be confused with a latrine, which is constructed on a deep pit. Dry toilets can include a squatting plate or pedestal, with a smooth finished surface and a limited area to minimise soiling. Dry toilets can be owner-built, or bought on the market. A dry toilet can be made from ferro-cement, fibre-enforced materials, or strong and durable plastic, painted wood and ceramic material.

Applying conditions
- Dry toilets should only be used in rural areas where sufficient space is available at the household level for storage, treatment and use of excreta.
- Dry toilets are suitable in water-scarce, flood prone regions, and on solid soils.
- The system is preferably used with anal wiping (using paper, leaves, grasses, etc. for anal cleaning). However, it can also be used in combination with a special anal washing facility. Washing water should be collected separately as in the Philippines. (See also the next description on 'dry urine diversion toilets').

Costs:	Unreinforced concrete squatting plate (mass production)	US$ 11 (Mozambique, 1995).
	Concrete squatting plate (based on 40 units)	US$ 9 – 11 (Niger, 1999).
Advantages:	**Disadvantages:**	
No water required for flushing.	The toilet has to be cleaned without using much water.	
Easy to construct with local materials.	Collected excreta have to be handled carefully, as they contain pathogens.	
May be used indoors.	Excreta have to be removed frequently, especially if the toilet is in the house.	
Information:	General — www.ecowaters.org	
	Toilet seats — www.riles.org	
	Squatting plates — www.sanplat.com	

Dry toilet pedestal in Mexico (photo RILES).
Insert: 'SanPlat' (about 1m^2) (photo www.sanplat.com).

Toilets

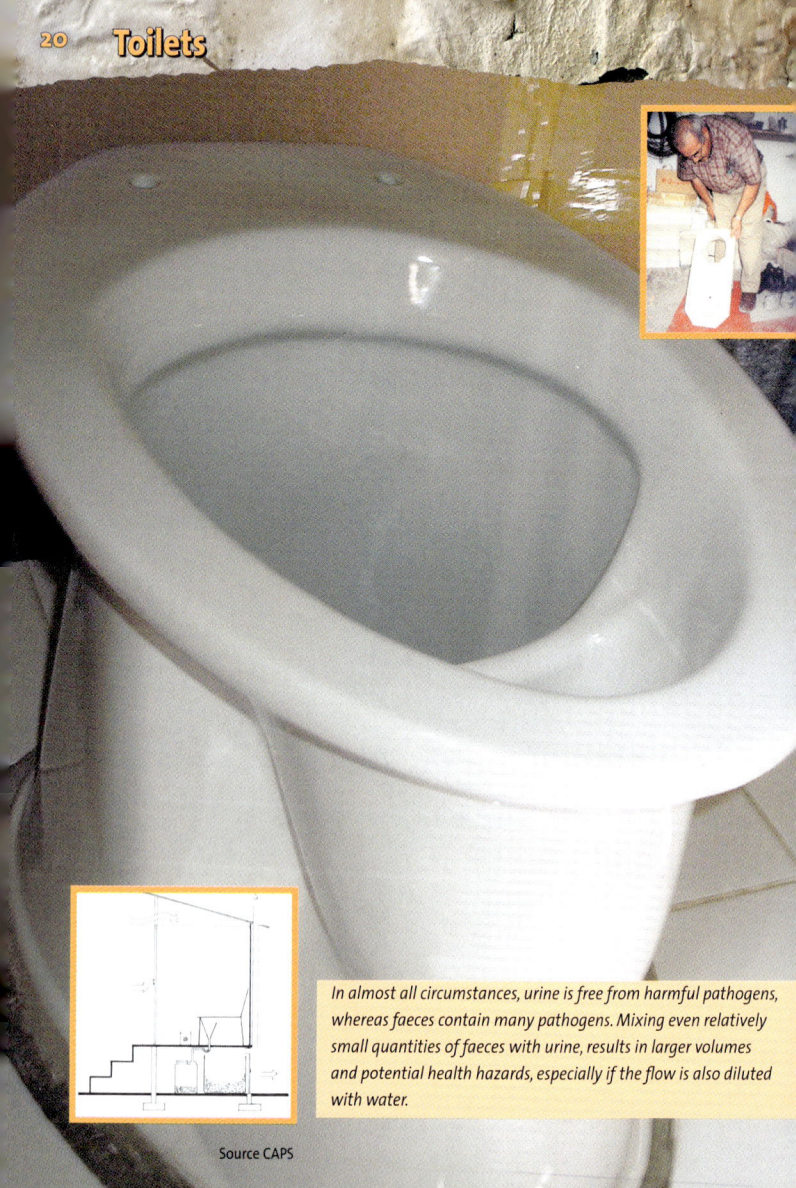

In almost all circumstances, urine is free from harmful pathogens, whereas faeces contain many pathogens. Mixing even relatively small quantities of faeces with urine, results in larger volumes and potential health hazards, especially if the flow is also diluted with water.

Source CAPS

Dry urine diversion toilets

"We have realised that the old latrine smells and has lots of flies, but the urine diversion system does not have these problems."
Thomas, son of a chief in the Chihota district in Zimbabwe.

The toilet has two compartments, keeping urine and faeces separate. Urine leaves the toilet through a pipe / tube. Faeces are stored directly beneath the toilet. After defecation, dry soil, ash or sawdust is spread over the faeces, controlling odour and absorbing moisture. Men, as well as women, need to sit while urinating to ensure that the urine is diverted into the correct channel.

Water used for anal cleaning must be kept separate in order not to dilute faeces or pollute urine with pathogens. This requires a separate facility for anal cleaning. Small amounts of anal cleaning water can be infiltrated. Larger volumes need to be treated (together with grey water) to prevent ground water pollution.

Dry urine diversion toilets can be made out of ceramic, ferro-cement, fibre-enforced materials, or strong, durable, plastic and painted wood. It is important that the surface is smooth and hardened.

Applying conditions

- Dry urine diversion toilets are used in regions that are water scarce, flood prone, or that have an impermeable and a high ground water table.
- They are suitable in rural and suburban areas, where urine and faeces can be used in agriculture.
- There needs to be sufficient public awareness about the risks of handling urine and faeces.

Costs:	Fibre glass pedestal (based on 20 units)	US$ 40 (Philippines).
	Ceramic pedestal (based on 400 units)	US$ 14 (Philippines).

Advantages:
The public health risks are mainly limited to proper handling of faeces.
Large scale nutrient recovery is a realistic possibilty.
Can be used indoors.
Does not require water for flushing.

Disadvantages:
Special child seats have to be provided to keep their urine and faeces separate.
The toilet's operation requires clear instructions and close attention.
Regular removal of collected urine and faeces is required.

Information:	General	www.gtz.de/ecosan
		www.ecosanres.org
		www.ecosan.nl
	South Africa	www.csir.co.za

Urine diversion pedestal with washing area in the Philippines (photo CAPS).
Insert: Urine diversion squatting pan in Palestine (photo WASTE).

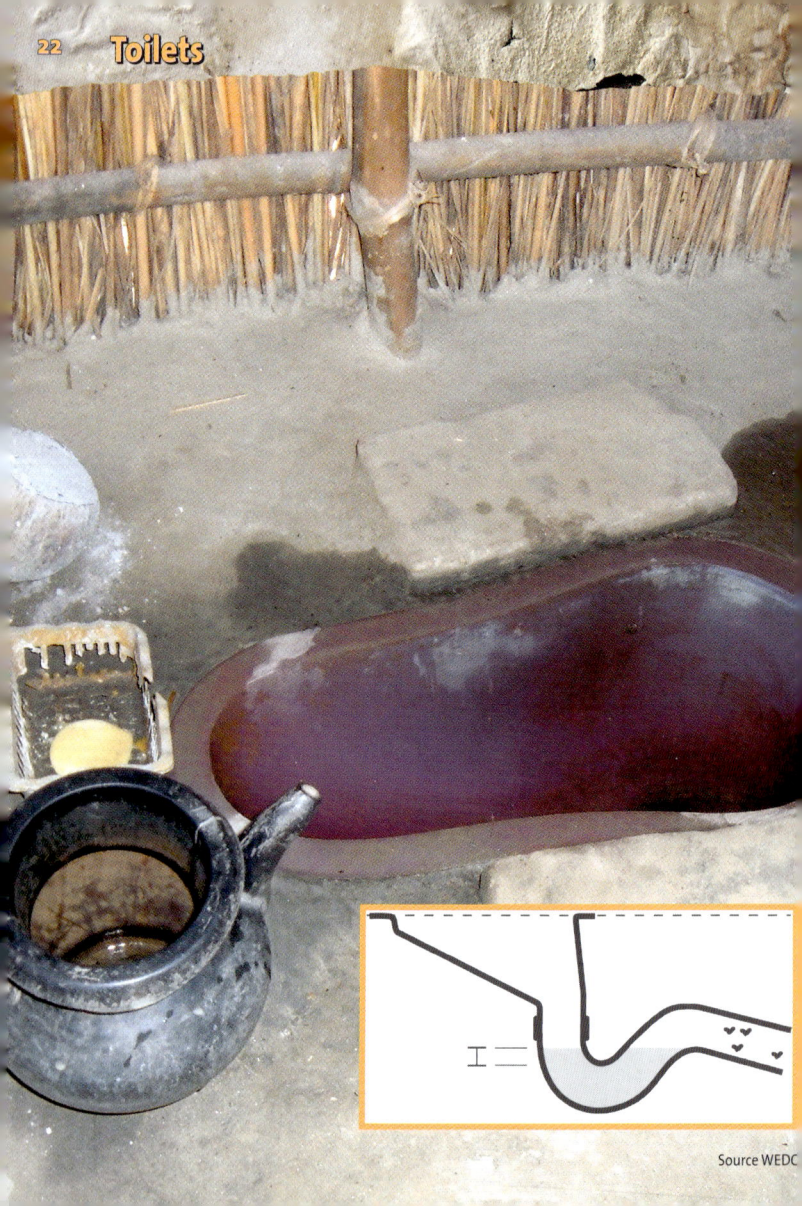

Toilets

Source WEDC

Pour flush slabs

Pour flush slabs (squatting pans) have a U-shaped facility partly filled with water under the slab. This U-trap overcomes problems with flies, mosquitoes, and odour by serving as a water seal. After use, excreta is manually flushed by pouring water into the pan with a scoop. About 1 to 4 litres of water is required for each flush. The amount of water required depends mainly on the design of the toilet and U-trap. Toilets can be made from plastic and ceramic, or from galvanized sheet metal.

Note: The principle of pour flush slabs can also be applied to the faeces compartment of urine diversion toilets.

Applying conditions
- Pour flush slabs can only be applied in regions where water is available for flushing, and the infrastructure is available or can be built to manage wastewater. This may require the construction of a (septic) tank / biogas digester / pit and / or small diameter sewerage.
- These slabs are especially appropriate in densely populated areas where dry handling of excreta isn't socio-cultural appropriate.
- Pour flush slabs are suitable where people use water for anal cleaning and squat to defecate.
- No material that should obstruct the U-trap should be thrown in the toilet. Bulky material used for anal cleaning can't be flushed through the U-trap.
- The U-trap should be checked monthly for blockages.

Costs: Ceramic pour flush pan — US$ 4- 8 (Tamil Nadu, India, 1999).
'Easyflush' polypropylene pan — US$ 2 (Chennai, India).
Maintenance costs — No expenses usually, except for the cost of the water.

Advantages:
High level of convenience for the user.
The design reduces the need to handle fresh excreta.
Can be used indoors.

Disadvantages:
The U-trap can easily become blocked.

Requires small amounts of water for flushing.

Pathogens are mixed with water and thus spread over a relatively large volume.

Information: General
www.who.nl
www.irc.nl
www.wsp.org

◁ **Low cost pour flush slab, Rajshahi, Bangladesh** (photo WaterAid Australia).

24 Toilets

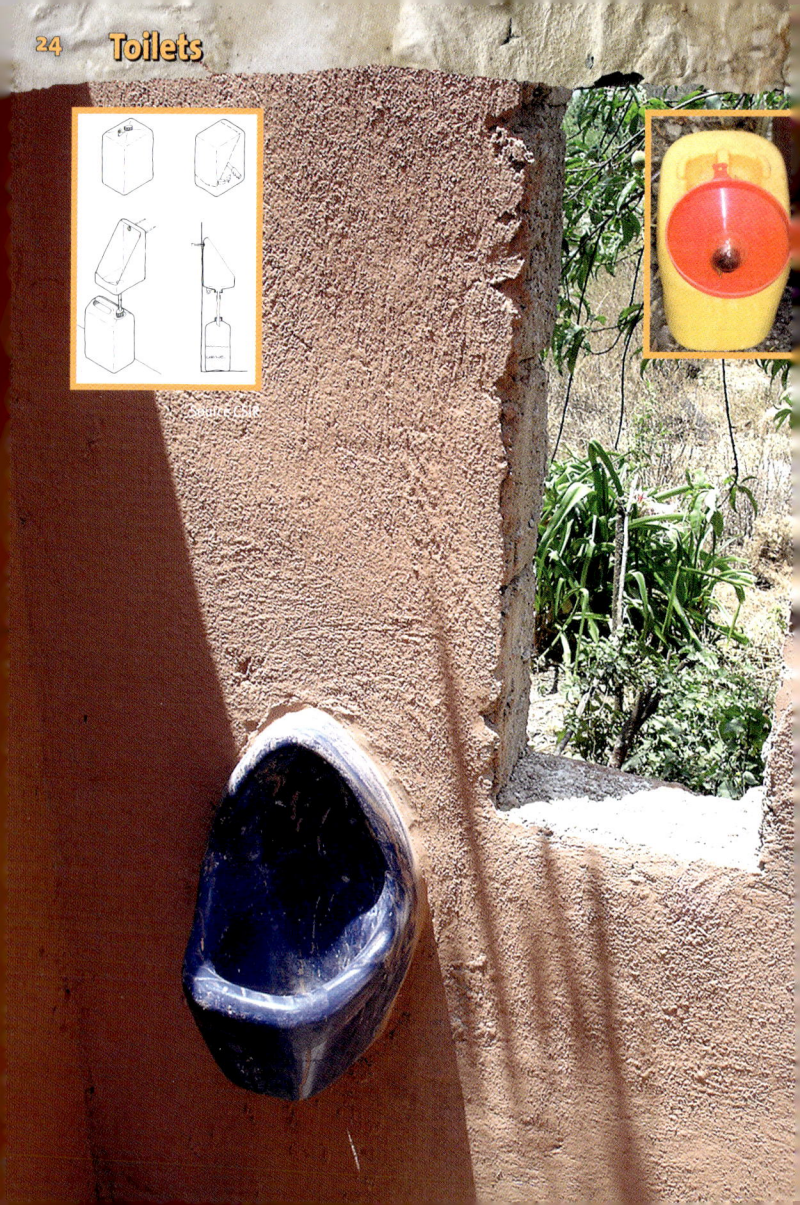

Waterless urinals

Waterless urinals, slab or wall-mounted, collect undiluted urine, and so generate relatively low volumes. Traditionally urinals are provided adjacent to a toilet. Urinals can prevent fouling of toilets, especially in schools.

Prefabricated urinals are available, but do-it-your-self toilets can also be made. The *'Eco-Lily'* from Ethiopia is made out of a common liquid container with a used light bulb acting as a floating 'odour-lock' to reduce smells.

The *'Eco-Lily'* is a device to be used as urinal both by men and women.

SUDEA's experiences have showed that men can use it without any explanation while women often need some information on how to use it because of their biological difference.

Applying conditions
- Waterless urinals are a suitable option in situations without reliable water supply.
- Urinals are a low-cost option, especially in public places where people use the toilet more for urinating than for defecation.
- Waterless urinals are often used in combination with a urine diversion toilet as the urinal allows men to urinate standing up.

Costs: Wall-mounted, manufactured urinal US$ 35 (South Africa).
Self constructed urinal Negligible.

Advantages:
Reduce water use.
Hygienic and cheap method for containing urine.

Disadvantages:
Doesn't deal with defecation.
Not useful for females.

Information: General www.schoolsanitation.org
www.irc.nl
Mexico www.laneta.apc.org/esac
East Africa http://user.tninet.se/~gyt516c/
South Africa www.csir.co.za
Ethiopia sudea@ethionet.et

▸ **Wall mounted urinal, Mexico** (photo WASTE).
Insert: *'Eco-Lily'* in Ethiopia (photo SUDEA).

Collection

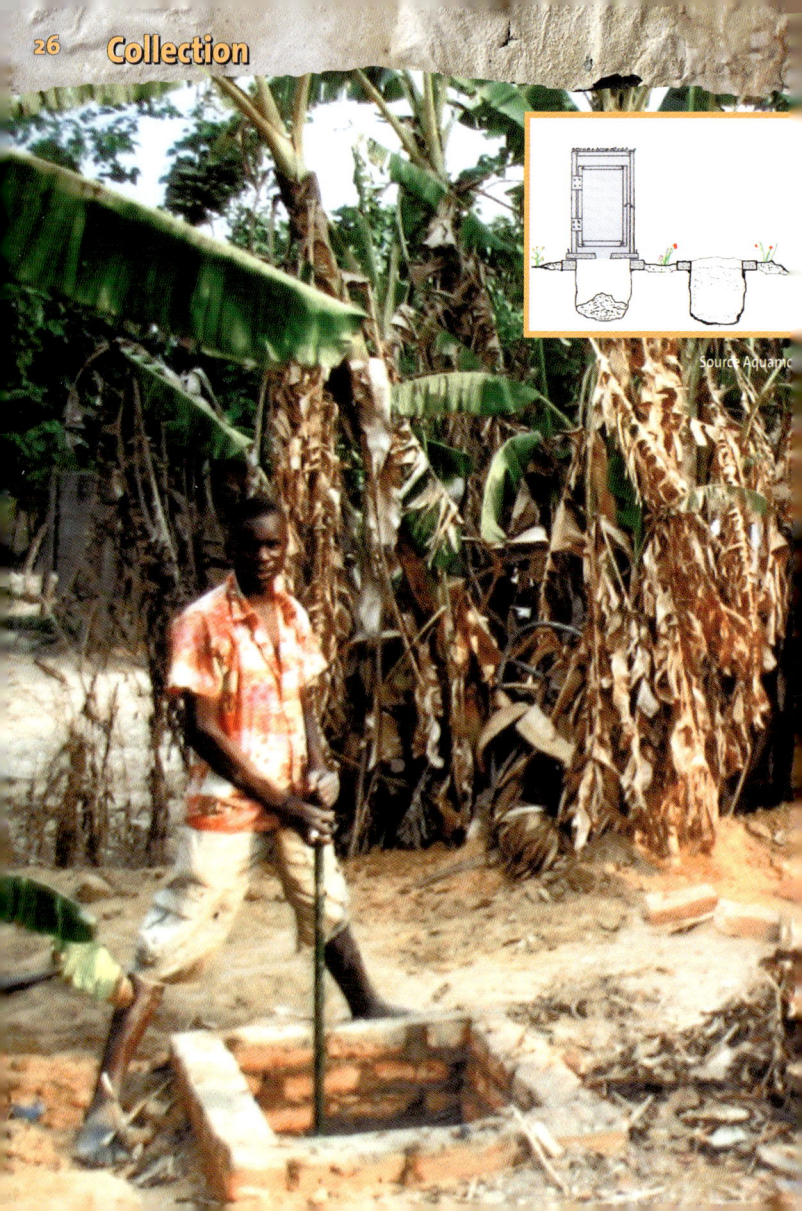

Fossa Alterna

The *Fossa Alterna* is a shallow alternating double pit system, collecting and composting excreta from a dry toilet. Two shallow pits are dug next to each other (0.5 – 1.5 metre deep). Dry leaves are added to the pit base before use, and thereafter soil (and ash) are added after each defecation. When a pit is 3/4 full, the concrete slab and portable superstructure are placed on the second pit. Excreta is not only collected, but also (pre-) treated by filling the original pit with soil and leaving it to compost. By the time the second pit is full, the first pit is emptied after which the slab and superstructure is put back on top of it and the pit is reused. After composting, the content of the first pit can be used as fertiliser. The best compost time is more than 12 months. The material can be excavated earlier at 6 months, but is best transferred at this stage to a pit in which a tree will be planted.

Family size
Small / medium sized
10 users

Capacity
About 0.5 – 0.75 m^3
About 1 m^3

Filling time
6 – 12 months
6 months

Applying conditions
- The conversion of excreta into humus will not take place if the pit is flooded with water. Therefore, the pit should not be sealed and water used for anal cleaning should not enter the pit.
- Not applicable in areas with a high water table, with very loose soil (which could collapse), or very solid soil which would prevent drainage.
- In order to prevent water tables penetrating the pits and contaminating the water, pits should be shallow.
- Applicable in rural and peri-urban areas, where compost can be taken away and disposed of or, better still, used on agricultural fields.
- As with many sanitation systems, household members need to understand the key principles for efficient operation and maintenance and discipline is required for adding soil after each defecation.

Costs: Construction of total system, including material and labour   About US$ 20 - 30 (Mozambique).

Advantages:
The design reduces the need to handle fresh faecal material.
Shallow depth of pit required.

Disadvantages:
No full recovery of nutrients.
Space required.
Cleaning of the toilet must be done with small amounts of water.

Information.   General   www.wateraid.org
                    Zimbabwe   http://aquamor.tripod.com

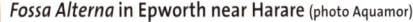

Fossa Alterna in Epworth near Harare (photo Aquamor).

Collection

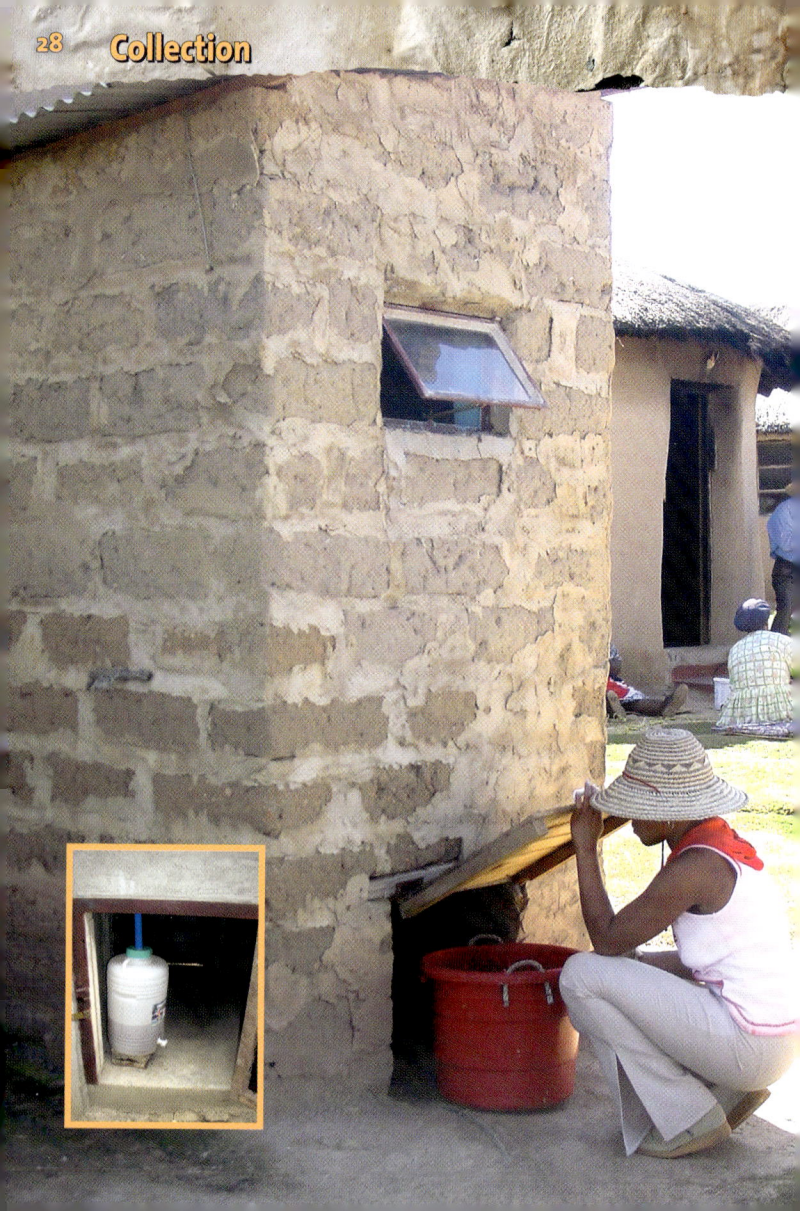

Oil drums and containers

Urine from urine diversion toilets or urinals can be collected in plastic containers. Oil drums are useful for the collection of faeces.

Urine collected in small containers (up to 20 litres) can be easily transported and used as fertiliser in the household's own vegetable garden.

Larger containers, filled with urine have to be collected by a vehicle and can therefore be transported over longer distances. Oil drums, or half drums, can be placed directly beneath a toilet to collect faeces. Ash or other drying material has to be added regularly to prevent smells. Toilet paper can also be collected in the oil drum.

	Family size	Capacity	Filling time
Container, polyethylene collecting urine	7 users	About 20 litre	2 days
Oil drum, polyethylene collecting faeces	7 users	20 – 100 litre	1 - > 5 weeks

Applying conditions
- Oil drums and containers can be used in areas with hard sub surface and high ground water tables.
- Not suitable for the collection of mixed urine and excreta.
- Collection of oil drums and containers at community level has to be made functioning beforehand and measures have to be taken to guarantee hygienic safety. Sizes and weights must be manageable.

Advantages:
Used oil drums and containers are available locally.
Adjustable to any size of logistic operation.

Disadvantages:
Handling of fresh faeces causing potential health risks.
Collection of mixed excreta not appropriate. Water used for anal cleaning should be collected separate.

Information:	General	www.gtz.de/ecosan
		www.waste.nl
	The Philippines	www.caps.ph
	India	www.sulabhinternational.org

◁ **Container collecting faeces in Uganda (photo J. Masondo, IRC).**
Insert: Plastic containers used for collection of urine in Mexico (photo WASTE).

30 Collection

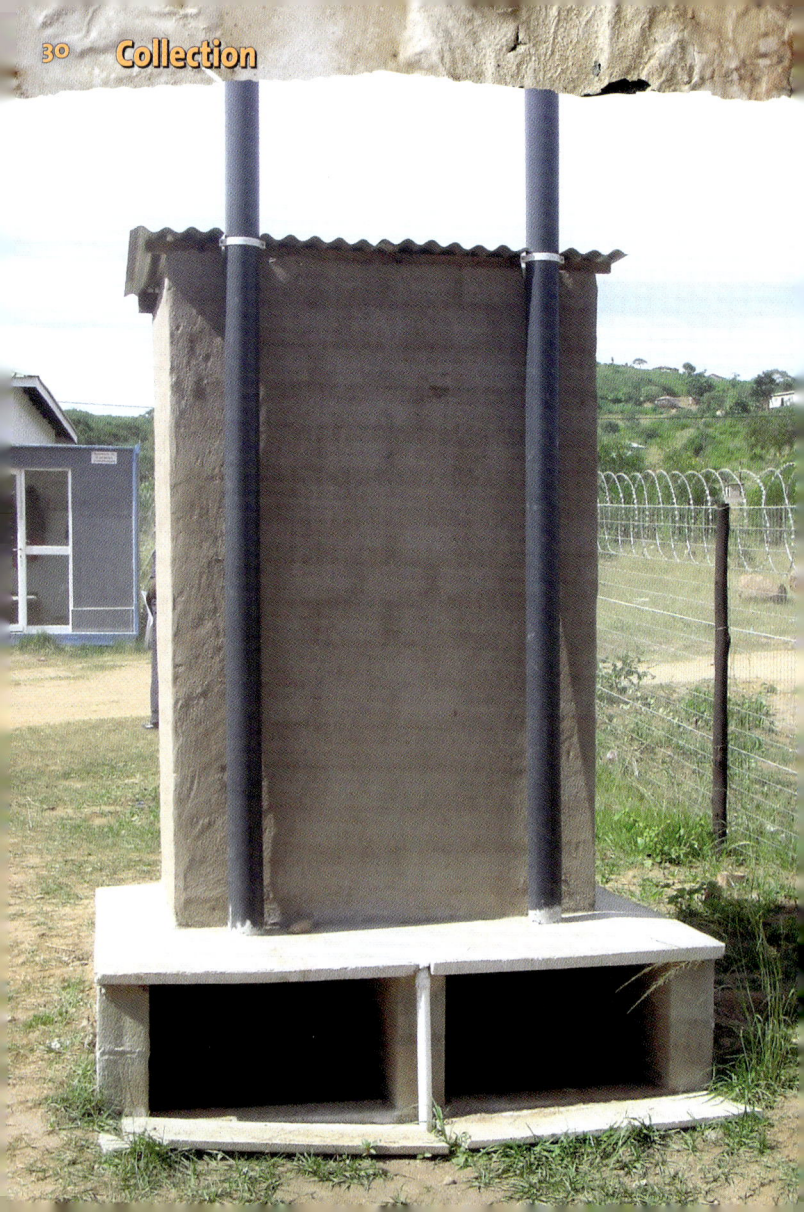

Vaults and chambers

Excreta from dry toilets and faeces from urine diversion toilets can be collected in vaults and chambers, built above ground, using bricks or stones, and accessible through a door. The floor should be made watertight from impermeable material. Excreta is not only collected here, but also (pre-) treated by pre-composting. Most systems use two chambers, in order to avoid handling fresh material; while one vault is filling up, excreta in the other vault is processed. These systems are referred to as *Double Vault systems*. For dehydration processes in these vaults, see Section Treatment – Dehydration, page 41.

Applying conditions

- Vaults and chambers are suitable in areas with a hard subsurface and high ground water table.
- The system can be applied in rural, as well as in urban areas. However, it should be noted that, if composted and dehydrated matter cannot be used on site, the need for transport will increase the operation and maintenance costs.
- Processing mixed excreta is only possible in arid climates.
- As with other dry sanitation options, the health risks related to handling of (pre-) treated excreta or faeces have to be taken into consideration.

Family size	Capacity	Filling time
7 users	0.6 - 0.8 m³	About 6 months

Costs:		
	Complete double vault system, freestanding unit	US$ 160 (Mexico, 1998).
	Complete double vault system, within the home	US$ 35 (China, 2002).
	Operation and maintenance	Negligible.

Advantages:
The design reduces the need to handle fresh faecal material.
On site pre treatment of excreta or faeces.
Relatively large emptying intervals.

Disadvantages:
Treatment process in the vault needs attention.

(Post) treatment of the excreta / faeces is required after collection.

Information:	General	www.who.int
		www.gtz.de/ecosan
	South Africa	www.csir.co.za
	Australia	http://www.enviro-options.com.au

◁ **Double vault system in South Africa** (photo J. Masondo, IRC).

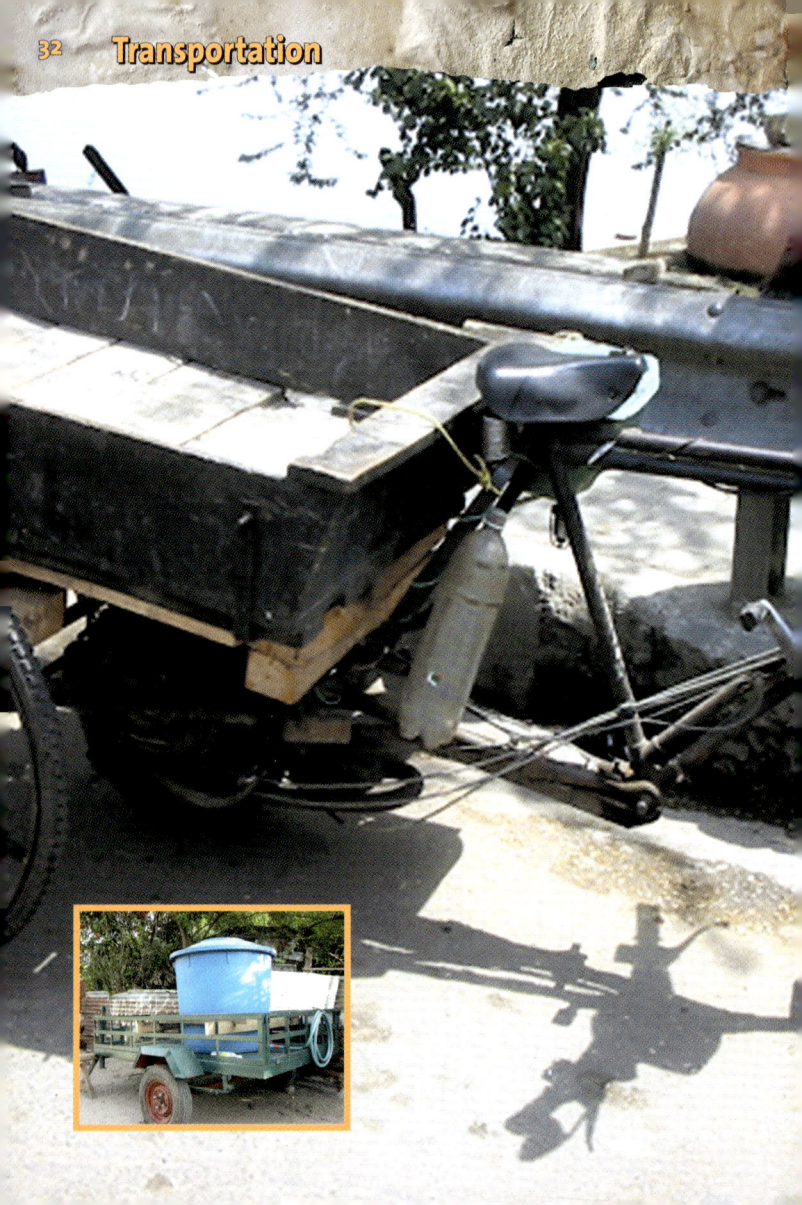

Cartage system

Tricycles and push carts can be used to transport containers and oil drums containing urine or excreta. Push carts and tricycles (pedal or motorised) can access small streets. Tricycles can speed up the collection operation and increase the radius of the collection in urban areas, transporting the containers to transfer stations or to community treatment facilities. From transfer stations, urine and excreta can be loaded onto trucks or tractors, which can haul a larger volume over a long distance. Tricycles can collect door to door, although urine can also be collected in larger containers serving a number of houses.

Applying conditions
- Pushcarts and tricycles are especially appropriate in flat urban areas, with access roads.
- Pushcarts and tricycles are not appropriate for collecting large volumes (> 300 litre, > 300 kg) or for longer distances.
- Operators require training and regulation.

Costs: Investment costs motorised tricycle — About US$ 300 (India, 2005).
Yearly operation and maintenance costs for the collection of faeces of 8000 households with motorised tricycles (incl. labour costs). — About US$ 2000 (India, 2005).

Advantages:
Not dependent on large, cost-intensive infrastructure.
Source of income for small private entrepreneurs.
Potential to link with solid waste collection services.

Disadvantages:
Highly depending on willingness to pay for regular removal of excreta.
Only appropriate for small haul distances and small volumes.
Transfer facilities often required.

Minimising operation costs may lead to uncontrolled disposal of sludge or urine.

Information: General
www.waste.nl
www.bpdws.org
www.sulabhinternational.org

◁ **Motorised tricycle in India** (photo WASTE).
Insert: Vehicle transporting urine in the Philippines (photo WASTE).

34 Transportation

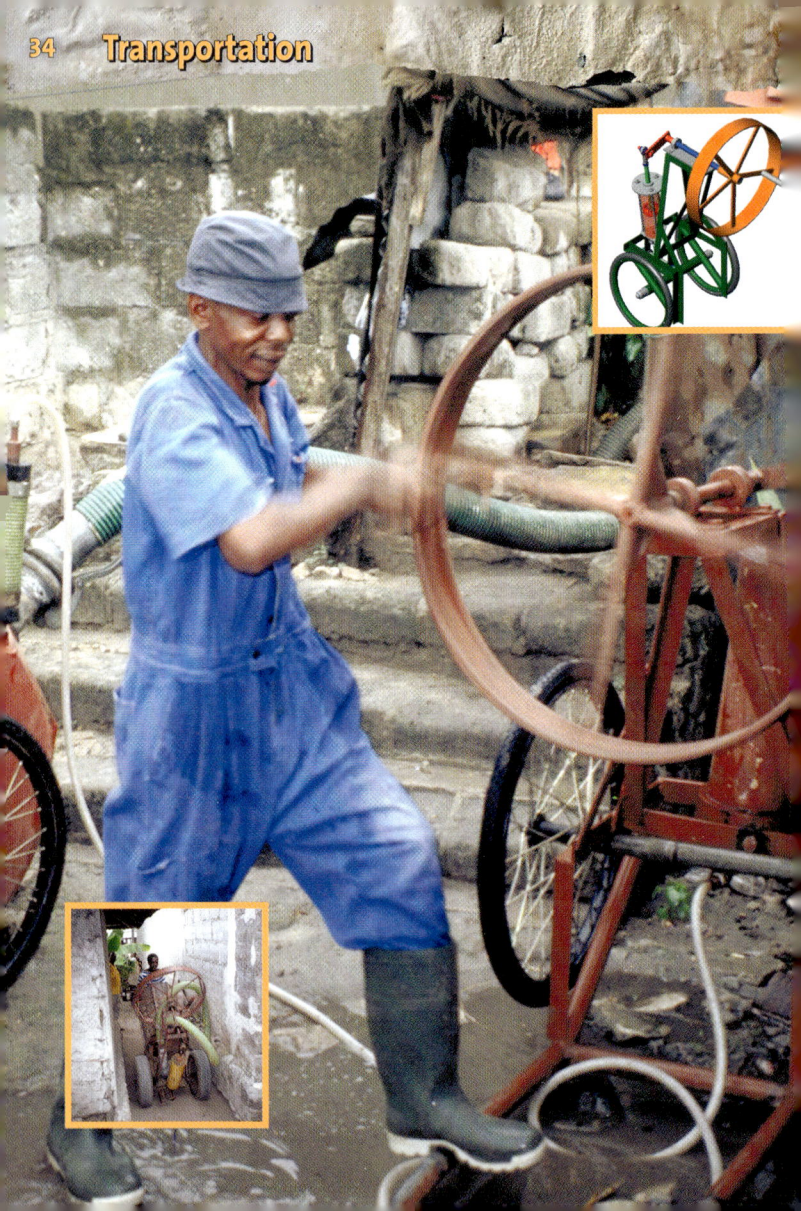

MAPET and Vacutug system

MAPET and Vacutug are two of the many more examples of mechanical emptying systems to empty pits and (septic) tanks. MAPET and Vacutug devices rely on informal or small scale, private operators to empty pits and (septic) tanks by means of mini-tanks and hand or motor operated pumps.

Both the Manual Pit Emptying Technology (MAPET) and the UN-Habitat Vacutug devices consist of a tank, a pump and flexible hosepipe. MAPET relies on a hand pump, which can fill a 200 litre vacuum tank in 5-20 minutes. The Vacutug consist of a 500 litre vacuum tank and a pump run by a small gasoline engine that has the capacity to remove sludge (or urine) at 1,700 litres a minute. MAPET equipment is mounted on a pushcart. The Vacutug is a small vacuum tanker with an engine that also powers the vehicle. Sludge is transported to a neighbourhood collection / disposal point from where vacuum tankers transfer it to city treatment plants.

Applying conditions

- Vacutug and MAPET technologies can be used to transport excreta in high-density areas with small-unpaved streets. Although designed to empty pits and septic tanks, these devices can also deal with urine.
- Operators require training and regulation.
- The system depends on a communal approach and economy of scale in order to allow these options to be sustainable.
- Wherever mechanised emptying is considered, the designs of the pits or (septic) tanks themselves should also be considered.

Costs:
	Investment MAPET	US$ 3000 (1992, Tanzania).
	Capital costs Vacutug	US$ 5000 (1998, Nairobi).
	Operation costs MAPET	US$ 2.50 /200 litre (1992, Tanzania).
	Operation costs Vacutug	US$ 3-5 / 500 litre (1998, Nairobi).

Advantages:
Low operation costs.
Can be constructed, operated and maintained using local materials and skills.
Capital cost are affordable by entrepreneurs who can develop micro-enterprises.

Disadvantages:
Solids are often not removed from pits or tanks.
MAPET is not suitable if the haul distance exceeds 0.5 km.
Minimising operation costs may lead to uncontrolled disposal of sludge or urine.

Information: General   www.waste.nl
Vacutug   www.hq.unhabitat.org
http://staging.unchs.org/vacutug.asp

▶ **MAPET in narrow street in Tanzania** (photo WASTE).
Insert: MAPET technology in use in Tanzania (photo WASTE).

Transportation

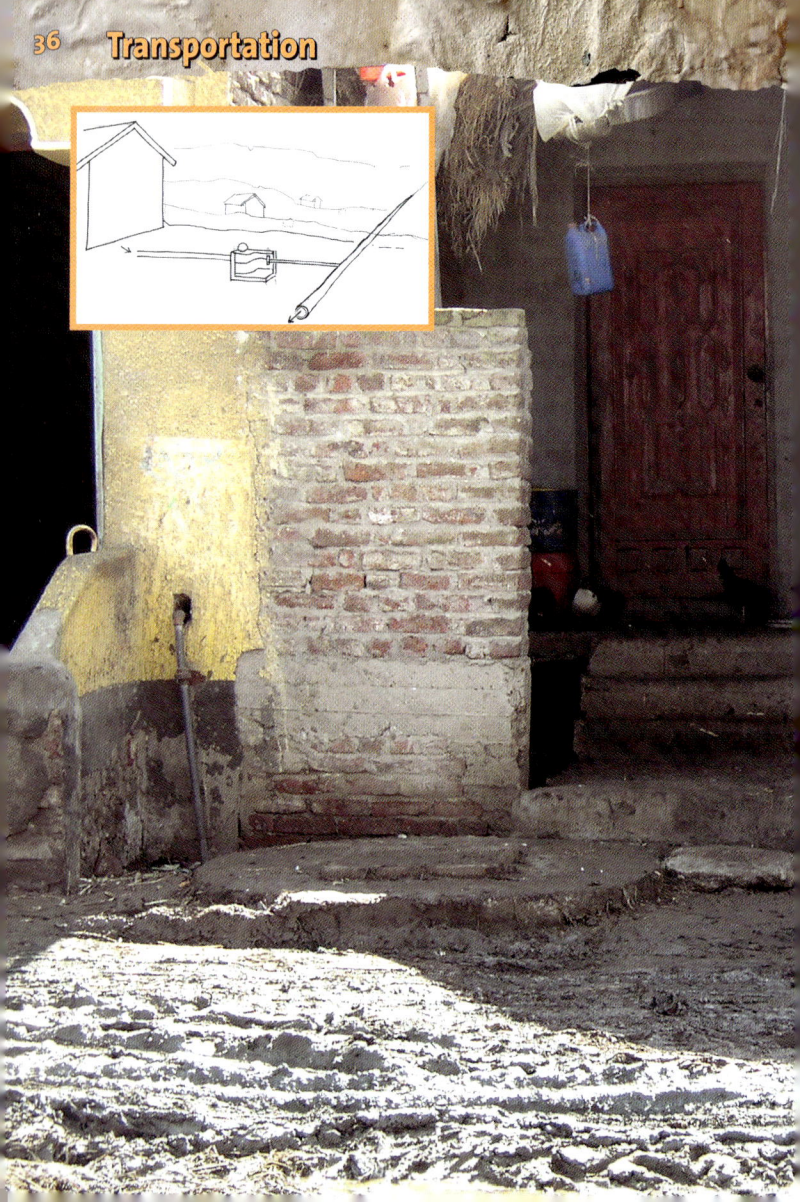

Settled sewerage (small diameter)

Settled sewerage, also called small diameter or small-bore sewerage is designed to prevent solids in wastewater from entering a communal small bore sewer network. An important condition for the functioning of these sewer networks is that a minimum average of 25 litres per person per day enters the system. First wastewater settles in a small interceptor tank. Later, wastewater is conveyed via small (50 – 200 mm) diameter sewers of PVC or other durable material. Pipes are laid at various gradients from 0% to 10%. Inspection manholes are limited to minimise unauthorised opening and disposal into the system. Costs can be reduced if a group of households shares one interceptor tank. Although settled sewerage is mainly used to transport wastewater, small diameter sewers are also appropriate to transport urine.

Applying conditions
- The system can be appropriate in high- and low-density areas.
- In areas where elevation differences do not permit gravity flow, pump stations are required.
- The system is appropriate for areas where septic tanks already exist, but effluent is causing public health or environmental risks.
- Understanding of the system hydraulics is required.
- The system needs to be flushed periodically to avoid blockages.

Costs:	Investment per household	US$ 150 – 500 (Honduras, 1990).
	Investment per person	US$ 35 – 85 (North East Brazil).
	Investment	20%-50% less than conventional sewerage in rural areas. Where septic tanks already exist, the cost reduction can be 40%–70% (USA).

Advantages:
Less dependent on active user involvement.
All kind of wastewater can be transported.
Little water needed to transport excreta through the small diameter pipe.
Sewers can be laid at flat gradients.
Excreta 'out of sight'.

Disadvantages:
Institutional operation and maintenance required.
Interceptor tanks need to be desludged periodically.
Potential risk of blockages due to illegal connections that by-pass the interceptor tank.

High water consumption for excreta removal.

Information:	General	www.sanicon.net http://www.efm.leeds.ac.uk/CIVE/Sewerage http://wedc.lboro.ac.uk

◀ **House with interceptor tank in a village in the Nile Delta, Egypt** (photo D. Mara).

Treatment

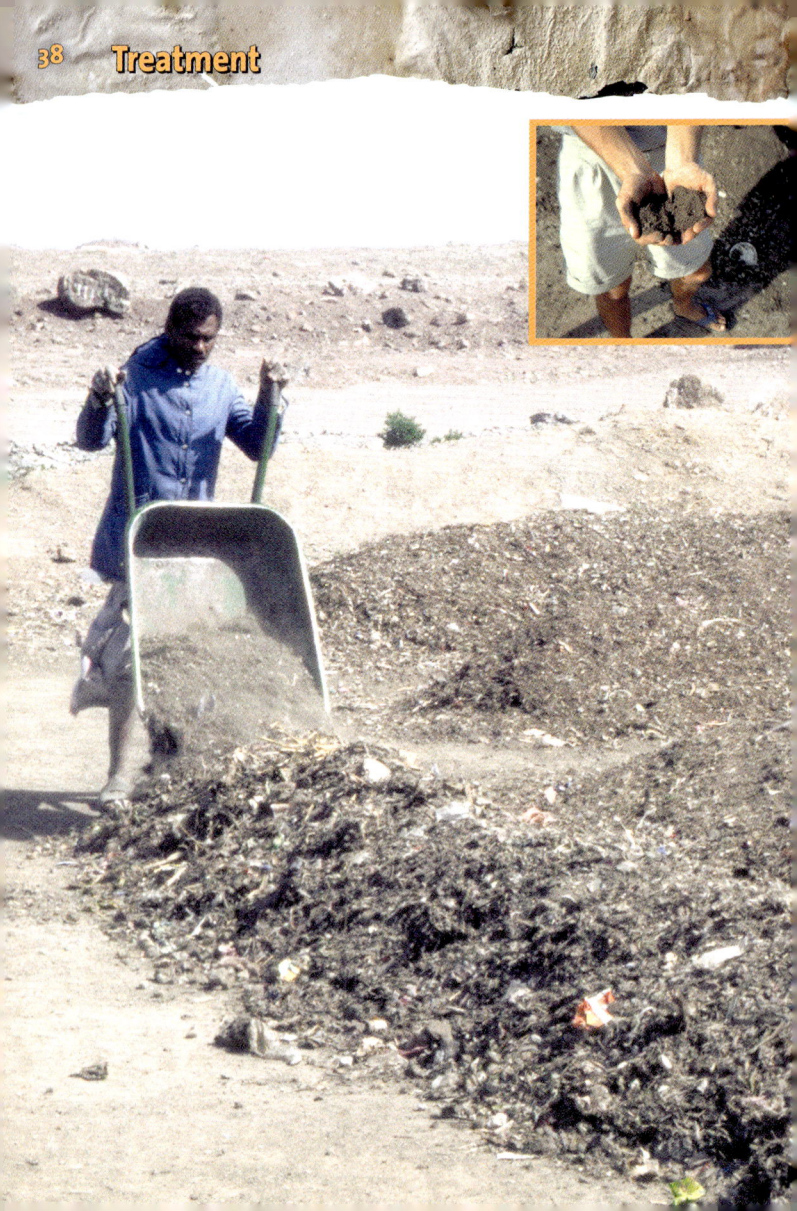

Co-composting

Composting is an aerobic process in which bacteria and other organisms feed on organic material and decompose it. Composting (one material) and co-composting (two or more materials) represent generally accepted procedures to treat excreta.

To start the composting process, the blended compostable material is placed in windrows (long or round piles). The 'recipe' combines high-carbon and high-nitrogen materials. Air is added to maintain aerobic conditions, either by turning the windrows or by forcing air through them. To adequately treat excreta together with other organic materials in windrows, the WHO (1989) recommends active windrow co-composting with other organic materials for one month at 55-60°C, followed by two to four months curing to stabilise the compost. This achieves an acceptable level of pathogen kill for targeted health values. Adding excreta, especially urine, to household organics produces compost with a higher nutrient value (N-P-K) than compost produced only from kitchen and garden wastes. Co-composting integrates excreta and solid waste management, optimizing efficiency.

Applying conditions

- The type of material, the climate, the amount of space and the equipment and funds available all influence the system design, especially windrow type and size, recipe, and level of technology.
- Special measures, such as more frequent turning or covering the piles can accommodate extremes of climate or temperature.
- Composting is a bio-chemical process, not a bio-mechanical one, and as such requires experience and practical knowledge, together with a high level of management.

Costs: Operation costs US$ 5 – 30/ ton composted material (costs are higher on smaller sites).
Capital costs Depend on scale, space available, and design choices.

Advantages:
Flexible approach with highly variable capacity.
Toilet paper is decomposed.
Through co-composting, a useful and safe end product is generated that combines nutrients and organic material.

Disadvantages:
Operation and maintenance requires moderate professional experience.
Limited control of vectors and pest attraction.
Lower cost variants have a high land requirement.

Information: General
www.ecosanres.org
www.gtz.de/ecosan
www.sandec.ch
www.waste.nl

Windrow composting in Yemen (photo WASTE).
Insert: Brazilian showing the compost (photo WASTF).

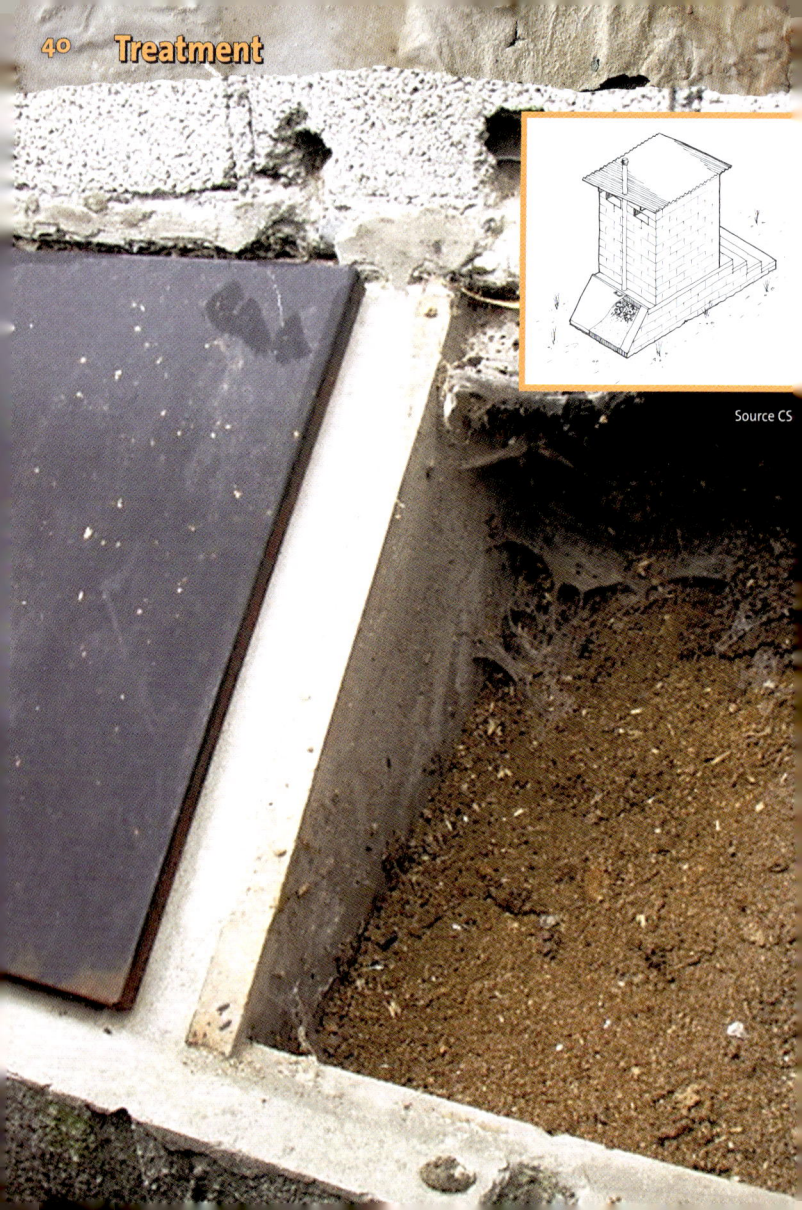

Source CS

Dehydration

In double vault dehydration systems, as described in the collection section 'collection' on vaults-chambers, excreta may dry inside the vault as a result of sun radiation, natural evaporation and ventilation. Absorbents such as lime, ash or dry soil should be added to the chamber after each defecation in order to absorb moisture, making the pile less compact. The product from a dehydration process is a kind of mulch, rich in humus, carbon, fibrous material, phosphorous and potassium. It should be stored, sun-dried or composted in order to kill off all pathogens.

Applying conditions

- Dehydration toilets are suitable in most climatic conditions, but function best in arid climates, with high average temperatures, long dry periods and short rainy seasons.
- Dehydration systems are most useful in rural and peri-urban areas, using the mulch onsite. Urban and large scale application has to be supported by collection systems. (See Section Transportation – Cartage system, page 33).
- Dehydration of excreta is favoured by diverting urine and anal cleaning water. Dehydrating mixed excreta only works properly in very dry climates.
- User commitment to operate and maintain the system is essential.

Costs:	Investment costs complete double vault system, freestanding unit	US$ 160 (1998 Mexico).
	Investment costs complete double vault system, in house unit	US$ 35 (2002 China).
	Operation and maintenance costs	Very low (no transportation included).

Advantages:	Disadvantages:
Efficient pre-treatment of excreta.	Poor maintenance can quickly lead to malfunctioning.
Maximum reduction of excreta volume.	Anal cleaning water should be kept separate.
Aesthetically acceptable end product.	

Information:	General	www.gtz.de/ecosan
		www.csir.co.za

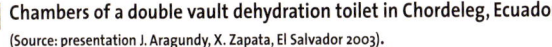

Chambers of a double vault dehydration toilet in Chordeleg, Ecuador
(Source: presentation J. Aragundy, X. Zapata, El Salvador 2003).

Treatment

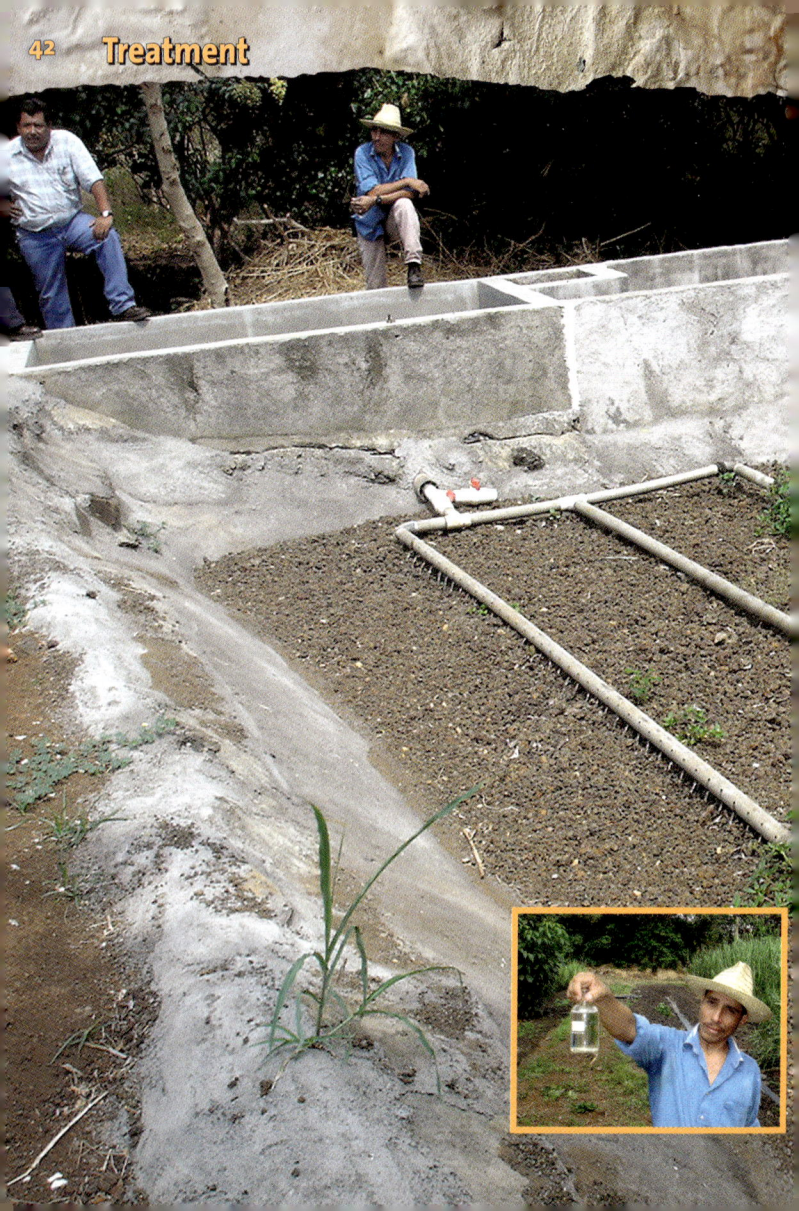

Planted soil filter

Planted soil filters, also referred to as constructed wetlands or reed bed systems, are natural systems treating solid-free wastewater. This can be pre-treated wastewater from a flush toilet or faecal wastewater from a urine diversion toilet, either combined with wastewater from the kitchen and bathroom, or separate from it. A planted soil filter, preceded by a settling and watertight storage tank, consists of a sand and gravel matrix (sealed at the bottom) planted with wetland plants like reeds. Solid free wastewater is discharged from the storage tank on top of the filter or though an underground inlet-system and flows through (vertical) the filter. Horizontal-flow soil filters are commonly found, and easier to construct than vertical flow filters, but they are less efficient at eliminating nitrogen. Wastewater is treated through several processes, in which bacteria play an important role. After treatment, the effluent can be discharged into surface water, used for irrigation or groundwater recharge.

Applying conditions

- If planted soil filters are applied in hot climates with a continuous growing season, wetland biomass can be harvested.
- Planted soil filters can be implemented at household or community level. Their use in isolated settlements like rural schools is also possible.
- Design and construction require a solid understanding of the treatment process.
- The amount of technical equipment needed is very small.

Costs can vary greatly, and depend, among other factors, on local availability of gravel, the kind of sealing and the cost of land.

Costs:		
	Investment costs on average	US$ 585 per person (Germany, 2005).
	Investment costs 7000 inhabitants	US$ 16 per person (Syria, 1999).
	Operational costs 7000 inhabitants	US$ 1.17 per person, per year (Syria, 1999).

Advantages:	Disadvantages:
Removes pathogens are from wastewater.	Considerably large area is needed for wastewater with high organic load.
Effluent from wetlands can be used for irrigation.	Some degree needed of post-treatment if the effluent is directly used for edible crop irrigation.
Operate without energy consumption.	Pre-treatment generates sludge.
Easy to operate. Intensive maintenance during first 2 years.	

Information:	General	www.bodenfilter.de/engdef.htm
		www.constructedwetlands.org
		www.gtz.de/ecosan
		www.sandec.ch

Construction of vertical planted soil filter in El Salvador (photo WASTE).
Insert: Treated wastewater in El Salvador (photo WASTE).

Treatment

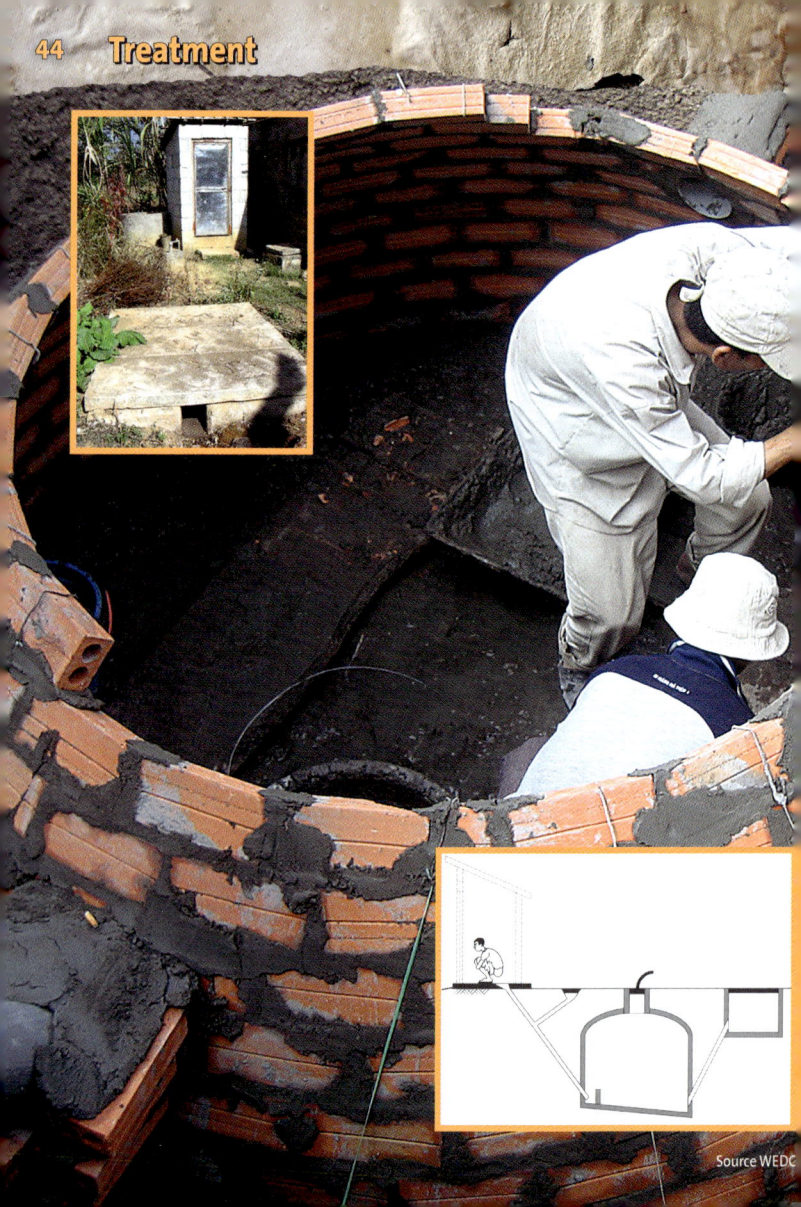

Source WEDC

Anaerobic digestion

In a digestion process, organic matter from human, animal or vegetable waste is broken down by microbiological activity, in the absence of air. This anaerobic process produces a combustible gas, methane, a source of (biogas) energy. The digestion process takes a couple of weeks to a couple of months after which the remaining slurry can be removed, either continuously or batch-wise. Several options are available, ranging from simple digestion techniques to technologically complex designs on a household or municipal scale. A domestic anaerobic digestion technique 'fixed dome type' consists of a simple biogas tank with a flat bottom and a round chamber covered with a dome shaped concrete gasholder. The gas is captured in the upper part of the digester. Gas pressure increases with the volume of gas stored, pushing the slurry into a separate outlet tank (see illustration).

Applying conditions

- Digesters are best suited to warm climates.
- They are most appropriate in rural areas where animal manure can be added to the process.
- The digestion process is sensitive to both temperature and materials. Both need to be controlled.
- Relatively high skills are needed for construction. Operation and maintenance, however, are simple for batch systems.

Investment costs vary greatly depending on the overall plant concept. Costs for biogas production increase with decreasing climatic temperatures. Life expectancy ranges from about 20 - 25 years.

Costs:	Investment domestic biogas plant in Nepal, (fixed dome types from 4 – 20m^3)	US$ 300 – 400.
	Maintenance costs (8m^3 digester)	US$ 5.50 – US$ 8.50 per year.
	Operational costs	Negligible.

Advantages:	Disadvantages:
Excreta 'out of sight'.	Gas safety risk.
Net production of clean renewable biogas.	Slurry from digesters has to be removed and treated.
Elimination of visual contaminants (e.g. toilet paper).	Insufficient pathogen removal without appropriate post treatment of sludge.
Low need for operational control and maintenance.	

Information:	General	www.itdg.org
		www.snvworld.org
		http://www5.gtz.de/gate/techinfo/biogas

◁ **Construction of biogas plant in Vietnam** (photo SNV Netherlands Development Organisation).
Insert: Outlet tank of biogas plant in Vietnam
(photo SNV Netherlands Development Organisation).

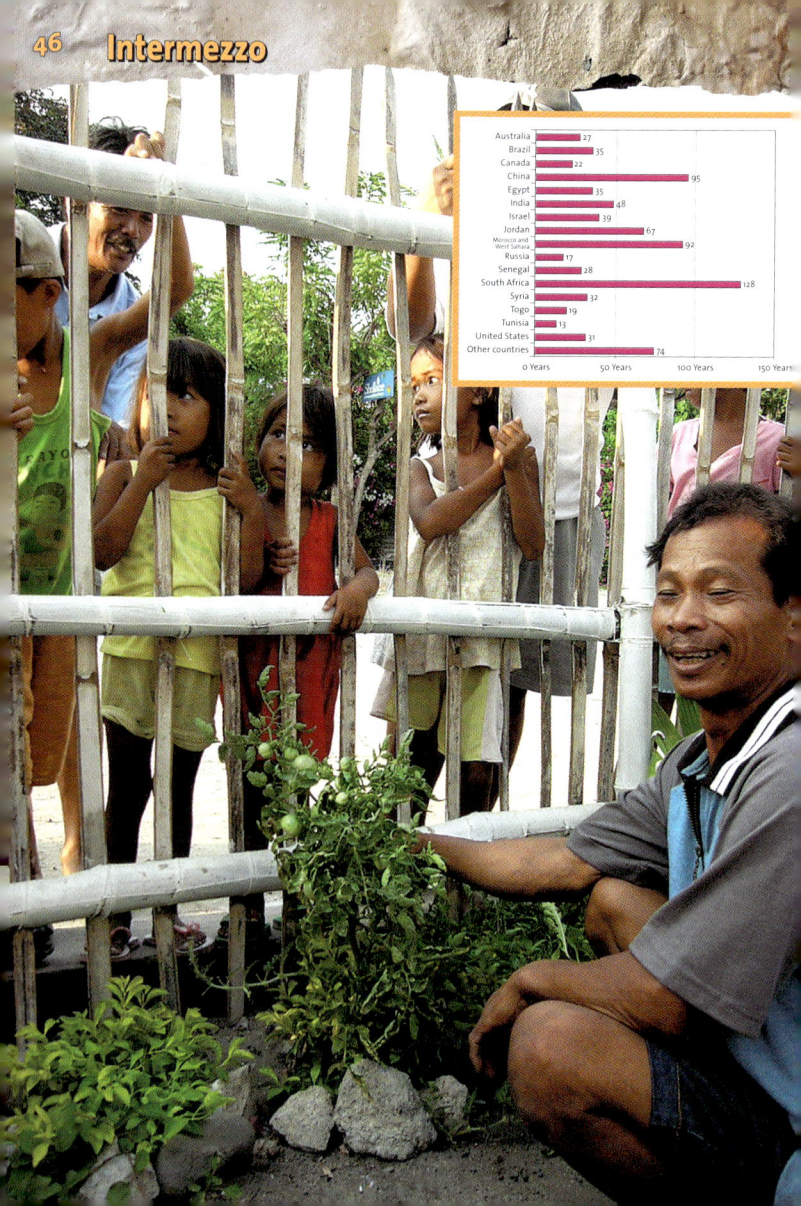

The need to recover phosphorous from excreta

The use of excreta and wastewater in agriculture is a daily occurrence, although it is rarely planned. Water and nutrients are recycled through crop production, and in this way sanitation contributes to food security and can improve household income and nutrition. There is much to be done to protect the health of farmers and the public from the potentially harmful effects of using human excreta and wastewater in agriculture, but with careful handling the process can be made safe, and there are many benefits.

Especially urgent is the need to conserve phosphorous. Annually, about 40 million tonnes of mined phosphorous is used to produce artificial fertilisers, needed for intensive agricultural practices in order to feed our cities.

The largest known sources of phosphorous today are in Western Sahara/Morocco and in China. Estimates of world supplies indicate that, at current rates of consumption, reserves will be exhausted within 150 years or less. Depletion will be faster if demand for phosphorous increases as expected, in which case reserves in many phosphorous exporting countries are likely to be exhausted within 30 years.

A complicating factor is that mineral phosphorous contains traces of cadmium. If cadmium levels are too high, it has to be removed, increasing the cost of mined phosphorous.

The most important causes of phosphorous depletion are inefficiencies in agricultural practices and the dispersal in sewage and solid waste of phosphorous contained in food and phosphate based detergents. Recycling phosphorous from topsoil requires slash-and-burn practices and is not a viable route. Recycling from sanitation and solid waste can be a partial solution. Radical changes in terms of source separation, recycling and containment of this scarce resource will be needed soon. In the light of this level of urgency, the absence of phosphorous from the discussion about sustainable global development is alarming. The need to recover phosphorous from excreta will become crucial for future generations!

Information: General
www.sei.se
www.fao.org
http://minerals.usgs.gov/minerals

Use of human urine in the Philippines (photo WASTE).
Insert: Phosphate rock: years of extraction remaining based on current reserves from 2005 using a 2% yearly increase (Source: SEI).

Using sanitation products

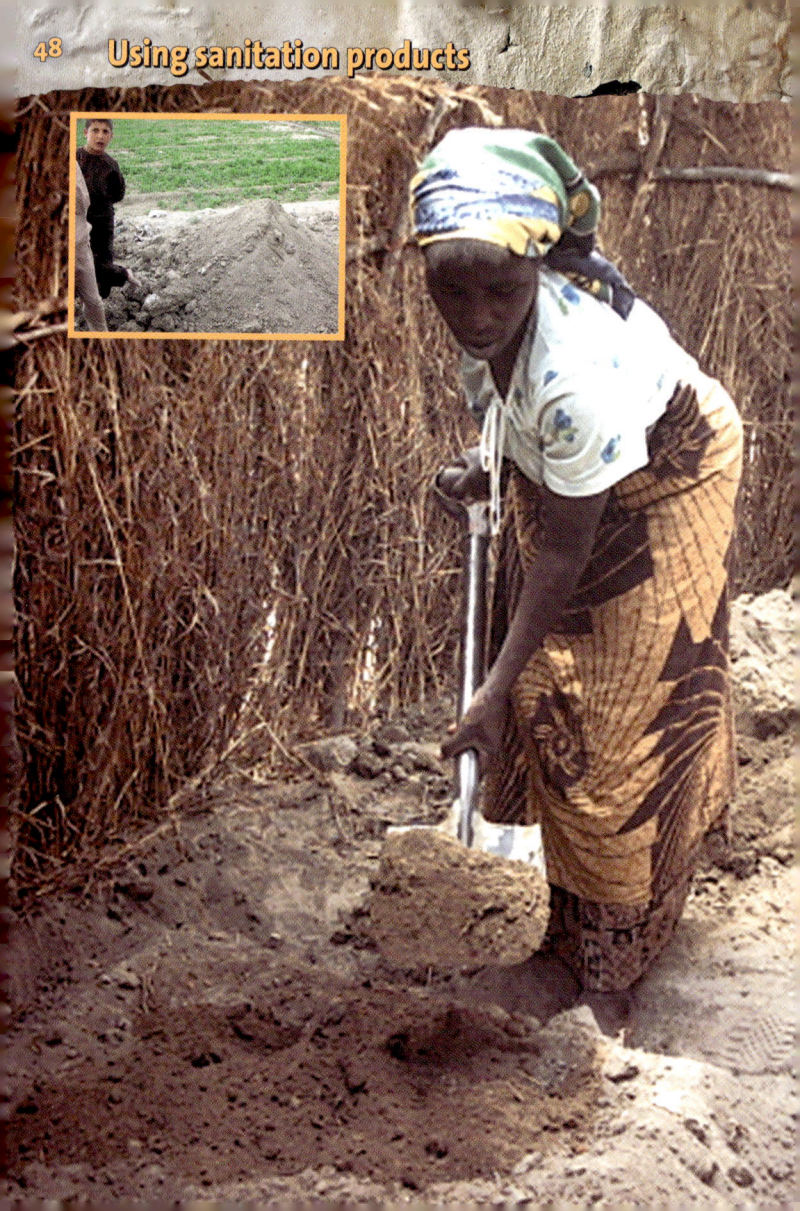

Compost as soil conditioner

"I got more yield by using compost. This year I have got beans and fibrous vegetables double in quantity than last year." (when he used chemical fertiliser)

From: Quazi, A.R. [NGO Forum for DWSS] Study on the re-use of excreta in Bangladesh. In: Environmental Sanitation Case studies to be published by IRC International Water and Sanitation Centre.

Decomposed excreta is rich in nutrients (NPK – nitrogen, phosphorous, and potassium) and organic material. The organic material in compost acts as soil conditioner. It also improves the structure and water holding capacity of sandy soils and adds structure and permeability to clay soils. Composted excreta, on its own or combined with other biodegradable material, enhances the fertility of topsoil.

Applying conditions

- Application of decomposed faecal matter at large scale is only recommended after full secondary treatment processes, meaning removal of all pathogens.
- Compost containing excreta should be applied before sowing or planting. The application rate can be based on the current recommendation for the use of phosphorous-based fertilisers.
- Compost containing excreta should be applied in such a way that the upper layer of the soil covers the material. Note; compost from excreta should not be applied as fertiliser to vegetables eaten raw.
- Personal protection equipment should be used when handling and applying the compost.

Advantages:
Compost reduces the need for artificial fertiliser.

Compost improves soil conditions.

Disadvantages:
Health precaution always needs to be considered when applying compost enriched with excreta!
Cultural taboos could hinder use.

Information: General www.ecosanres.org
http://aquamor.tripod.com

◁ **Using compost in a vegetable garden in Malawi** (photo Aquamor).
Insert: Application of compost as soil conditioner (photo H. Mang).

Using sanitation products

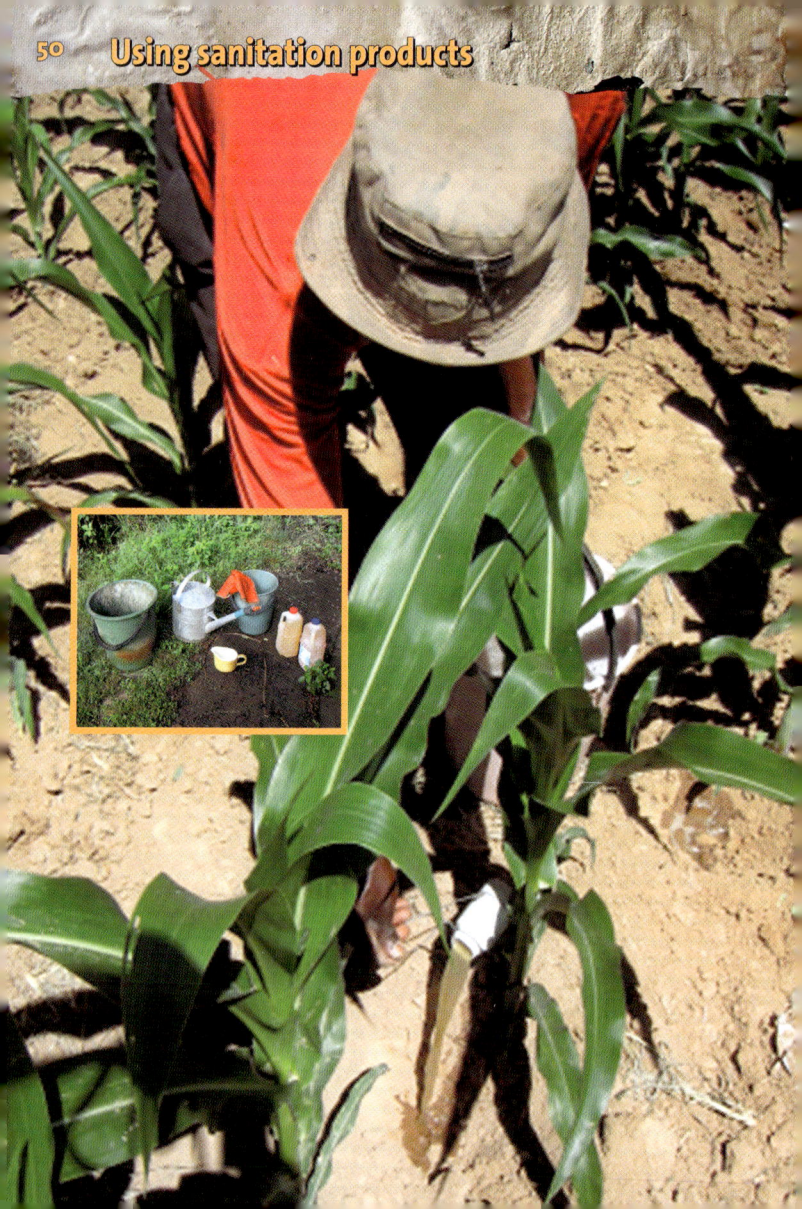

Human urine as fertiliser

When asked what she is growing with the urine and wash water, Nandawathi laughs and says, "Chillies, but we think we will only use them after drying, not fresh!"
Nandawathi, Matale Town, Sri Lanka.

Urine is a high quality, low cost alternative to the application of nitrogen-rich mineral fertiliser in plant production. The application of urine should be done as close to the ground as possible, incorporating it into the soil, preventing nitrogen loss. Urine is therefore preferably mixed with soil, or watered into it. The amount applied and the frequency of application depends on the nitrogen need of the plant and its root size. In general, recommendations available for the use of nitrogen fertilisers give a good starting point for how to use urine. The risk of disease transmission through handling and using human urine are related mainly to faecal cross-contamination.

For large-scale systems, storage times ranging from 1-6 months is recommended at ambient temperatures, depending on whether crop to be fertilised are eaten raw or cooked. Urine should preferably not be diluted before application to discourage microorganism growth, to improve the die-off rate of pathogens and to discourage mosquitoes from breeding.

At household level, urine can be used without storage, for all type of crops that are for the household's own consumption, so long as the crops are not harvested within a month of fertilisation. One reason for more relaxed guidelines for single households is that person-to-person transmission of pathogens outweighs the risk from fertilisation with urine.

Applying conditions
- Urine should not be applied in areas with high salinity.
- Recommendations for storage time and application techniques must be fully understood and followed.

Advantages:	Disadvantages:
Urine replaces mineral fertilisers. Nutrients are directly available to plants.	Large volume compared to artificial fertiliser. Health precautions needed when applying urine! Cultural taboos could hinder use of urine.
Information: General	www.smi.ki.se www.who.int www.ecosanres.org

◀ **Application of urine in a hollow next to the plant, Harare** (photo Aquamor).
   Insert: General equipment for applying urine (photo Aquamor).

Using sanitation products

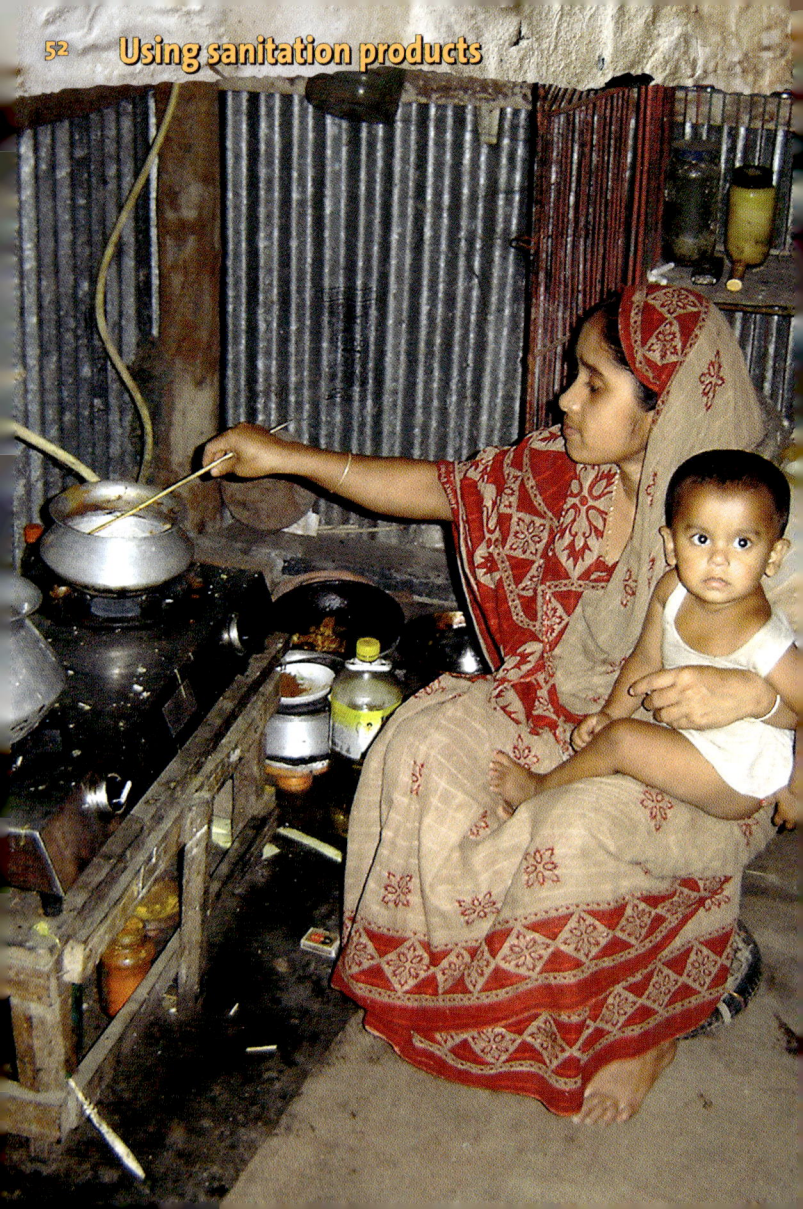

Biogas as source of energy

Ms Jharna, resident of Dhopagata village, and housewife of the family, informed that earlier she used to cook with kerosene and she was not comfortable with it as the operation and maintenance of the kerosene oven is difficult. Now she is enjoying cooking with biogas and she finds it as good as natural gas.
From: Quazi, A.R. [NGO Forum for DWSS] Study on the re-use of excreta in Bangladesh. In: Environmental Sanitation Case Studies to be published by IRC International Water and Sanitation Centre.

Biogas is a mixture of methane (60%) and carbon dioxide (40%), produced by anaerobic digestion of organic material, usually animal dung, human excreta and crop residue. Small-scale biogas digesters provide fuel for domestic lighting, cooling and cooking. Large-scale biogas plants are able to produce sufficient gas to fuel engines to generate electricity. The (thermal) energy available from biogas is about 6 kWh/m^3. This corresponds to half a litre of diesel oil and 5.5 kg of firewood. 1 kg of human faeces generates about 50 litres of biogas: 1 kg of cattle dung delivers 40 litres of biogas, and 1 kg of chicken droppings generates about 70 litres of biogas.

Applying conditions

- The main prerequisite of biogas use is the availability of specially designed biogas burners or modified consumer appliances.
- In some cases, especially at larger scale, further treatment or conditioning of biogas is necessary before it is ready to use. Treatment aims to remove water, hydrogen sulphide or carbon dioxide from the raw gas.
- Safety measures are needed, especially to reduce the risk of explosion in case of leakages.

Advantages:
Clean energy supply, reduces non-renewable energy use and decreases respiratory disease. Reduces workload in collecting firewood and in cooking. Deforestation and soil erosion can be reduced.

Disadvantages:
Biogas lamps have lower efficiency compared to using kerosene.

Information: General

www.snvworld.org
http://www5.gtz.de/gate/

Biogas used for cooking in Bangladesh (photo SNV Netherlands Development Organisation).

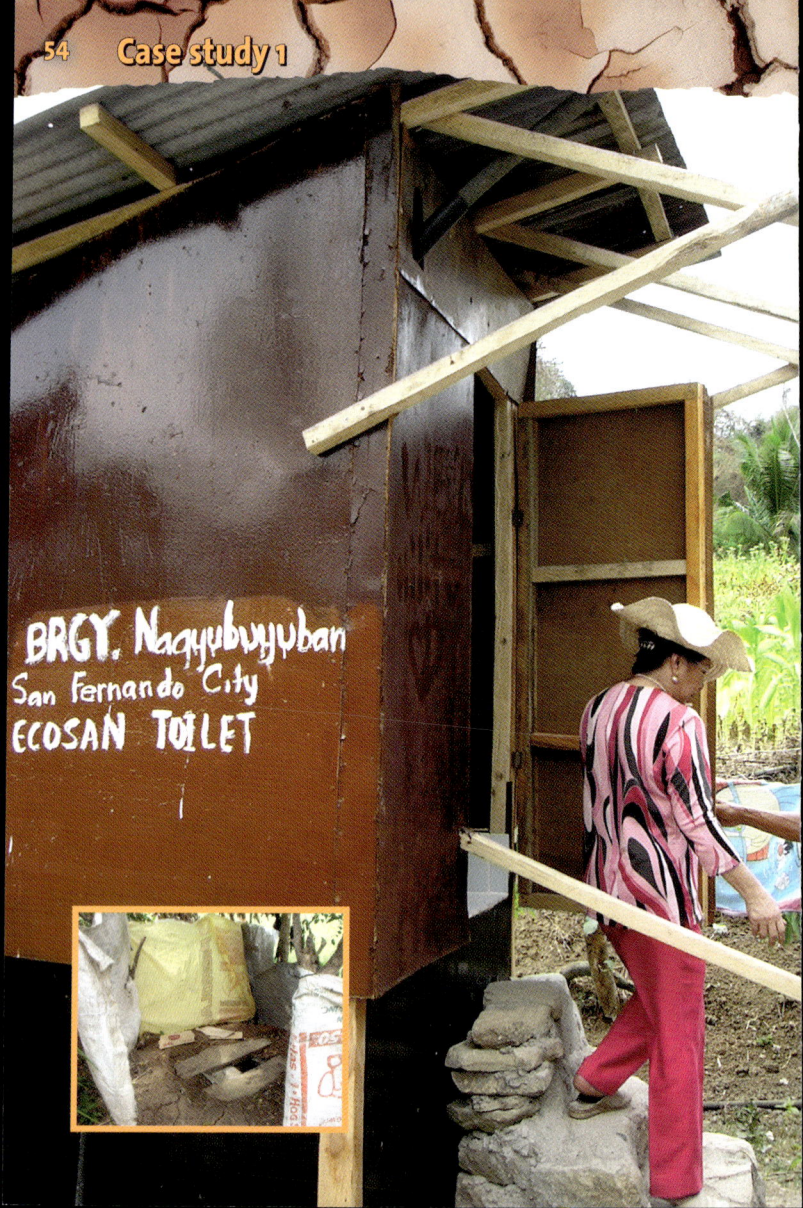

Case study 1

BRGY. Nagyubuyuban
San Fernando City
ECOSAN TOILET

Case study 1: Urine diversion in the Philippines

The initial situation

In the Philippines, about 30% of people lack access to improved sanitation. This figure varies from region to region and in San Fernando City in La Union Province, the proportion without improved sanitation is lower, at about 10%. This still approximates to 2,500 households, mainly in poor coastal barangays (villages) and remote uplands where people defecate in open fields, use open pits, or have access to unhealthy communal toilets. Poverty, ignorance about the consequences of poor sanitation and lack of awareness about alternatives, led to sanitation issues being neglected. As a consequence, many wells in the city are contaminated. Until 2004 in San Fernando, the only option for improving sanitation was to install pour flush toilets. These comprise squatting slabs connected to a septic tank, usually one per toilet, which needs regular emptying. Because the cost of the emptying service is relatively high, users often don't seal the bottom of the septic tank to allow seepage into the ground and so reduce the frequency of emptying. As a result, effluents pollute the environment and the shallow groundwater. In three of the coastal barangays, communal toilets facilities could not be properly used, mainly due to the unavailability of water for flushing.

Improving sanitation conditions

The city authorities became convinced that public health would only improve if all citizens had access to proper sanitation that did not pollute scarce drinking water resources. When the City Mayor, Mary Jane C. Ortega, read about ecological sanitation in December 2003, she decided to implement this in her city. Ecological sanitation involves recovering and reusing the resources contained in excreta and wastewater, and Mayor Ortega saw this as a way to empower the community, through a process of capacity building and social preparation that involved workshops, training and seminars at city, barangay and household level. Therefore, the Mayor decided to involve communities as agents of change, starting with two of the poorest barangays.

Smart sanitation

The technology: Within a year, two low-income barangays in San Fernando (San Augustin and Nagyubuyuban) had begun to install and use waterless (dry) urine diversion toilets. The toilet is sited 60-100 cm above ground level allowing faeces to fall into a collection container directly underneath. Meanwhile the urine runs off to a small liquid container. The substructure has a single chamber accommodating 25 litre container drums or a 50 litre plastic (HDPE) container, which can be easily transported when full.

◁ **The City Mayor visits the newly built toilet in San Fernando** (photo WASTE).
Insert: Sanitation conditions in San Fernando, before the new toilets were built (photo WASTE).

Appropriateness: Households collect the excreta themselves, using composted faecal matter and urine as fertiliser on their gardens or few acres of land. Carbonated rice husk, which is locally available, is added to the faecal matter to absorb moisture, improving the composting process and reducing odour to a minimum. A good ventilation pipe connected to the container chamber does the rest. Urine is collected in a 5-gallon plastic container outside the toilet. Water used for anal cleaning is collected separately in a special washing area and directly used to irrigate crops or bananas.

Implementation: People who install these toilets in their homes are known as ecological sanitation co-operators. Before construction begun, a series of seminars was organised, teaching co-operators about careful handling of faeces and grey wate and prepare them socially and technically to use and maintain their urine diversion toilets. The households joined a financing scheme through which they pay for the urine diversion toilet in instalments before the construction of the facility, while they were being trained. The city provided the substructure of the toilet. The co-operators provide the 'counterpart', in other words the roof and walls. This does not need to be expensive, co-operators use readily available local materials such as *nipa* or *sawali*, dried leaves of trees native to the Philippines.

Sustainability: The use of ceramic urine diversion toilets and arrangements for collecting urine and anal cleaning water, led to large amounts of urine and other liquid being collected. With the success of the scheme, the amounts became too large for family gardens in the coastal village of San Agustin. Co-operators became alarmed that 'watering' their plants with too much urine would harm the plants rather than make their harvest bountiful.

Every barangay or village in the Philippines is required to construct a Materials Recovery Facility or MRF for solid waste. The city had already decided to store partly composted human faeces in the MRF, and process it there to turn it into a useful fertiliser. To deal with the surplus of urine, a urine storage and treatment facility was developed at the San Agustin MRF, under the Philippines' Ecological Solid Waste Management Act. A local university department is investigating the potential for co-composting urine and organic municipal waste for agricultural purposes.

The narrow alleys of barangay San Augustin do not allow a door-to-door collection service, so households take their urine surplus each week to a central collection point. From there, a vehicle collects the urine into a large container on a small trailer and takes it to the MRF.

An ecological sanitation committee in each village, consisting of the barangay chief and other members, carries out coordination and management of the co-operators and the finance schemes. The urine collection service is arranged by the ecological sanitation committee in cooperation with city staff.

Tobacco growers and other large agricultural producers have been persuaded to substitute mineral fertilisers for human urine. In the upland rural barangay of Nagyubuyuban, the farmers directly use urine and faecal matter on the fields. The availability of land, the low cost of urine collection and familiarity with organic fertilisers, make this a sustainable practice.

Cost comparison

The costs vary depending on the materials used. For the case of San Fernando, readily available materials like native materials and recyclables (for the roofs and walls) were used to lower the cost of construction for the co-operators. The following cost estimates are based on the present prices of the materials in San Fernando City, La Union (February 2006). The prices are expected to increase in summer.

	W.C. (Reinforced concrete)	Urine diversion 1 (Flat sheets)	Urine diversion 2 (Reinforced concrete)
Materials:			
Concrete and masonry	617	18	164
Steelworks	81	35	44
Walls (flat / corrugated sheets)		12	
Windows (Jalousie glass window)	2		2
Doors (Plywood panel door)	47	13	47
Tiles	152	12	129
Toilet	49	20	20
Wash bowl		20	20
Urinal		6	6
Lavatory (hand washing)	19	19	19
Piping	20	23	23
Finishing works	23	14	23
Electrical works	13	13	13
Roofing	26	26	54
Containers	household	household	household
Labour	374	76	187
Estimated total investment costs	**US$ 1430**	**US$ 290–310**	**US$ 740 - 760**

Case study 1

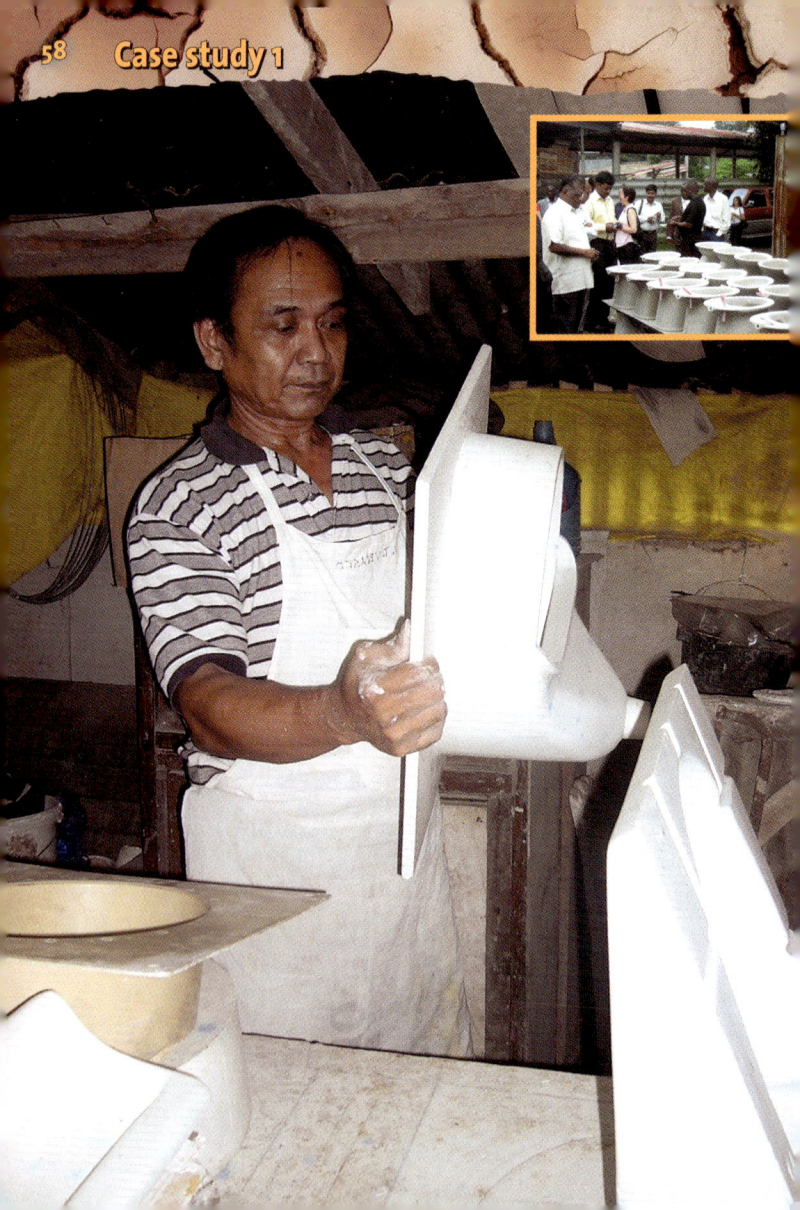

Scaling up

The decision to introduce ecological sanitation into two poor barangays appears to have been a key turning point in the city's sanitation strategy. Popularisation of the dry urine diversion toilet benefited from the city's attitude that this was not a second best solution but a powerful instrument to improve the community's health and wealth. Several local entrepreneurs were involved in the design of the dry toilet. Outsourcing production to local artisans and craftsmen contributed to their rapid introduction in San Fernando. As a result, the price and quality of locally made urine diversion toilets are equal to or better than those of similar products in the shops.

The city now integrates the concept of dry ecological sanitation into its strategic sanitation planning, under the slogan *Sanitation for All = A Healthy Environment for All*. As a result, there is an increasing demand for this new sanitation option among local communities.

Loans and micro credits schemes have been made available to small and informal enterprises who also benefit from becoming involved. Families receive financial incentives from a revolving fund.

As well as the City Mayor, the sanitation project has other local champions who will continue to support the scheme when the term of office is over for the current elected officials. Government regulations and national laws also encourage local government officials to put ecological sanitation on their agenda.

Information:	CAPS	www.caps.ph
	City of San Fernando	www.sanfernandocity.gov.ph
	WASTE	www.waste.nl

▶ **Production of urine diversion toilet moulds in the Philippines (photo WASTE).**
Insert: Mass production of urine diversion toilet in the Philippines (photo WASTE).

Case study 2

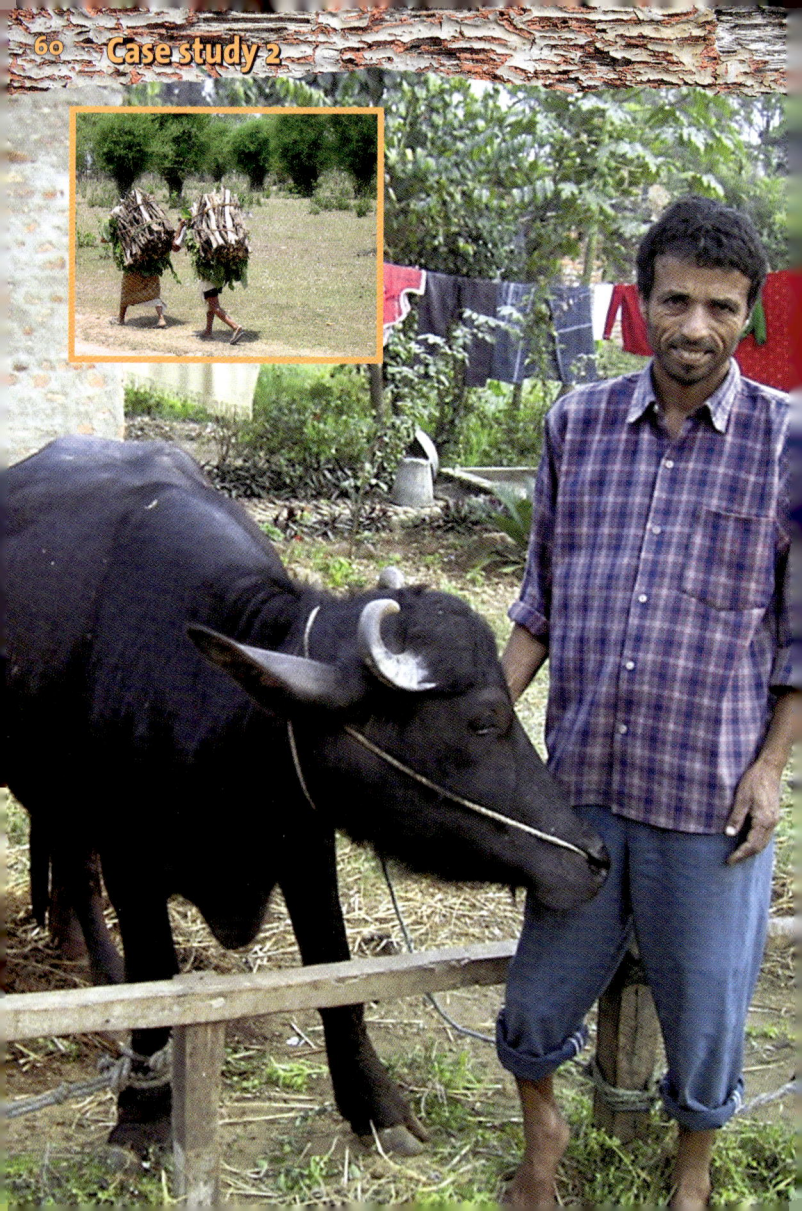

Case study 2: Fixed-dome biogas systems in Nepal

Biomass (organic matter) is by far the mostly commonly used fuel in the South. Biomass energy is derived from plant and animal material, such as wood from forests, residues from agricultural processes, and industrial, human or animal wastes. Biomass can be used directly (e.g. burning wood for cooking) or be converted into a liquid or gaseous fuel (e.g. ethanol from sugar crops or biogas from animal and human waste). Biogas is suitable for cooking, lighting and heating.

Other benefits are improved sanitation, reduced deforestation, inexpensive fertilisation, reduced water source pollution, clean air and reduced CO_2 emission.

Despite the great benefits of large-scale use of small-scale biogas technology, it is only widely applied in China (15 million domestic biogas plants[1]) and India (over 3 million domestic biogas plants[2]). Seeing these examples, Nepal started the introduction of this *Smart-Tech* at large-scale.

The initial situation

Poor sanitation: According to official sources, about 27% of the population has access to improved sanitation facilities in Nepal, (68% in urban areas but only 20% in rural areas[3]).

Deforestation: Wood, agricultural residues, and animal dung provide more than 80% of the total energy consumption for fuel In rural areas, this is even higher, at more than 95%. Wood is still the main source of fuel, resulting in serious deforestation around villages and increased soil instability on hillsides.

Health effects: The smoke from burning biomass waste has caused widespread eye and respiratory diseases with women and children.

Livestock: Cattle, water buffalo, poultry and other livestock play an important role in the lives of Nepalese farmers, and can guarantee a continuous source of fuel for biogas systems. Pour flush or flush toilets can be connected to these systems as additional feeders.

◁ **One big buffalo provides the dung required to operate the smallest sized biogas plant in Nepal** (photo SNV Netherlands Development Organisation).

Insert: Less fire wood collection needed in Nepal after introducing biogas plants
(photo SNV Netherlands Development Organisation).

---

[1] Mr. Wang Jiuchen, Director of Energy Ecology Division, Department of Science and Education of the Chinese Ministry of Agriculture, cites the number as 15 million domestic biogas plants as per December 2004.

[2] The Annual Report of the Ministry of Non-Conventional Energy Sources (MNES) of the Government of India, cites the number as 3.67 million domestic biogas plants as per April 2004.

[3] The Mid-term Assessment of Progress, 2004, Joint Monitoring Programme for Water Supply and Sanitation, WHO/UNICEF, 2004.

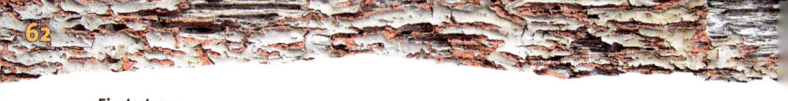

First steps

BSP: Although the first official biogas programme was launched by His Majesty's Government of Nepal in 1974, the installation rate of biogas plants remained low in the beginning until the early 90s. Then the Nepal Biogas Support Programme (BSP) was started with the main goal to promote the large-scale use of biogas as a substitute for wood, agricultural residues, animal dung and kerosene in rural areas. Although in name the programme achieved national coverage, it mainly reached farmers with above-average incomes who were comparatively accessible and who were accommodating towards the scheme. Many other farmers were not yet able to afford the initial cash payments.

Smart Sanitation

The fixed dome biogas system consists of the digester itself, a gasholder, an inlet, and a slurry outlet. Different sizes are available ranging from 4 to 20m^3 (4, 6, 8, 10, 15 and 20m^3). Dung, homogenised with water, is fed into the digester in quantities that depend on the size of the plant and the ambient temperature. At moderate temperatures, as in the hills of Nepal, the daily input amounts to 6kg of dung per m^3 of plant. Depending on the ambient temperature, the slurry will remain in the digester for 50 to 70 days. The gas produced is used for cooking and to a lesser extent for lighting (by 20% of users). At the end of this period, the slurry flows into a compost pit, from where it is returned to the fields as a fertiliser, to restore its remaining nutrients to the soil.

The small fixed-dome digester currently most in use can easily accommodate the attachment of a toilet, by including an additional inlet pipe, saving the cost of constructing separate sanitation facilities. Initially, strong cultural taboos restricted toilet connections to 10% of installations. Current figures indicate that 70% of biogas plants include toilet attachments.

Appropriateness

If a smallholder has at least two cows or buffalos and lives on own land below an altitude of 2.000 metres, a biogas digester of 4m^3 is already feasible. It is very appropriate because:
- The toilet is easy to use and to clean, and requires little or virtually no maintenance.
- Allows a toilet to be conveniently placed indoors.
- Contributes to a reduction in diseases caused by poor sanitation, to a reduction in respiratory infections and eye illnesses caused by smoke.
- Keeps water sources safer as it eliminates groundwater pollution.

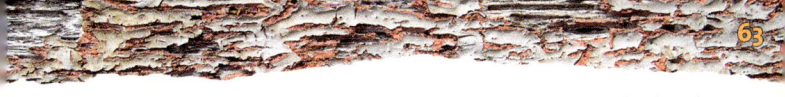

- Prevents further deforestation and soil erosion, and provides organic fertiliser for crops and trees.
- Reduces greenhouse gas emissions by about 4.6 tons of CO_2 equivalents per digester of $6m^3$ per annum.
- The technology can be easily replicated and locally made.
- It is, with the help of micro-finance and limited subsidies, affordable to many low-income people.

Sustainability

Many benefits for families. With a $6m^3$ digester a farming household saves about 3 tons of firewood and 38 litres of kerosene per year. Each household saves not less than 900 hours a year (2,5 hour per day!) because they have a reduced need to collect firewood and because cooking takes less of their time. Each biogas reactor supplies sufficient smokeless gas to cook the meals for one family.

The gains for society are equally great. On the environmental front, the use of biogas reduces deforestation and improves soil conservation. In social terms, it leads to better school attendance, and fewer illnesses. In economic terms, it generates employment and reduces economic losses due to poor health. Local resources, including materials, manpower and finance, can be deployed, helping to start a new industry and related businesses. It has been estimated that 11,000 new jobs have been created through BSP.

Implementation and scaling up

At the start of the programme, only one state owned company was producing biogas systems. Today, more than 50 private companies are producing such systems, meeting strict production standards in order for farmers to qualify for subsidies. Financial support in the form of a loan and subsidy programme targeting small and medium-scale rural farmers, was a critical element in developing the commercial market for biogas plants.

The operation and maintenance of a biogas system is the responsibility of the owner. Staff from the construction companies offer groups of new users a one-day-training on operation and management. Nearly 85% of the trained users are female.

Results

BSP has successfully commercialised and scaled-up the use of animal and human excreta as a renewable and sustainable energy source. Biogas plants have substantially improved the lives of rural smallholders, and of women and children in particular.

The following table summarizes some significant results. It shows that the size of farms implementing biogas solutions has fallen substantially, and that the number of households benefiting has risen accordingly. In the first 18 years only 70,000 people adopted this technology. In the succeeding 11 years a further 600,000 people began to benefit, and in the two years to 2005, another 180,000 joined, despite a decrease in subsidies.

Phase	1 (1974 - 1992)	2 (1992 - 2003)	3 (2003 - 2009)
Size of farms (averages)	8 cows 4.9 hectares	5 cows 1.3 hectares	3 cows 0.75 hectares
Households accumulated	11,000	111,000	141,000 (2005) 200,000 (target)
Total people accumulated	70,000	670,000	850,000 (2005) 1,200,000 (target)
Plant size	> 12 m^3 avg	1.2 m^3 avg (1992) 0.6 m^3 avg (2003)	< 0.6 m^3 avg
Subsidy	50%	27%	17%
Partners	One bank One company	4 credit-providers 50 companies 30 NGOs 3 donors	
Production	600 per annum	12,000 p.annum	17,000 p.annum
Focus	Development	Supply side	Demand side
Quality	Fair, bur erratic	Improved	ISO 9000 Level

Lessons learnt

A number of factors came together to make the development of this smart sanitation solution a success:

- 'Ownership' of the smart sanitation solution by the target group and main stake-holders has been a key factor in the overall success of BSP.
- Design was based on the real needs of the end user and addressed their concerns in a suitable, maintainable, repairable, safe, replicable and affordable way, geared to existing market realities.
- Programme concept was well understood and accepted by users.
- Direct and visible gains for each user, as well as clear societal gains.
- Development and use of local renewable resources and materials.
- Creation of opportunities for local business.
- Generation of employment.

- A stable enabling environment that embraced policy, incentives, finance, micro-credit and training.
- Commitment to securing involvement from the main financial, managerial, technical and political institutional stakeholders, and to building their capacity.
- Commitment to openness and financial transparency, so that Incentives for market development reached the target group rather than the manufacturers.
- Initial start-up investment necessary to bring the process to a point where it can be self-sustaining through a commercial, market approach.

Multiple benefits at household, local, national and global level
- Key benefits related to health, gender, environment and institutional capacity.
- Solution of a cluster of serious problems (no energy, deforestation, water source pollution) with a single smart solution that brought a range of social and economic benefits in one go.
- The formula not only achieved its primary aim, (clean energy) but also addressed the public good (forest conservation, clean air, employment).
- The monetary value of most of these benefits is not quantifiable. However, the financial and economic analysis of the costs and benefits that are quantifiable clearly demonstrate the value of biogas plants and the BSP: Return on Investment is good: for a 6m^3 digester, estimates vary from 16% to 21% for the financial internal rate of return (FIRR) and from 35% to 68% for economic internal rate of return (EIRR) (see table below).

Cost plant	6 m^3 size	$300 / unit
FIRR	Plain Tarai	21%
	Hills	16%
EIRR	Fuel savings	35% [4]
	+ Saved labour	41%
	+ Nutrients saved	53%
	+ Health benefits	56%
	+ Reduced carbon	68%
	+ Indirect benefits school attendance, children care, etc	> 70%

Information:	www.snvworld.org
	www.biogasnepal.org
	www.biogas.org.vn

[4] These EIRR figures are from 2003 Evaluation of BSP.

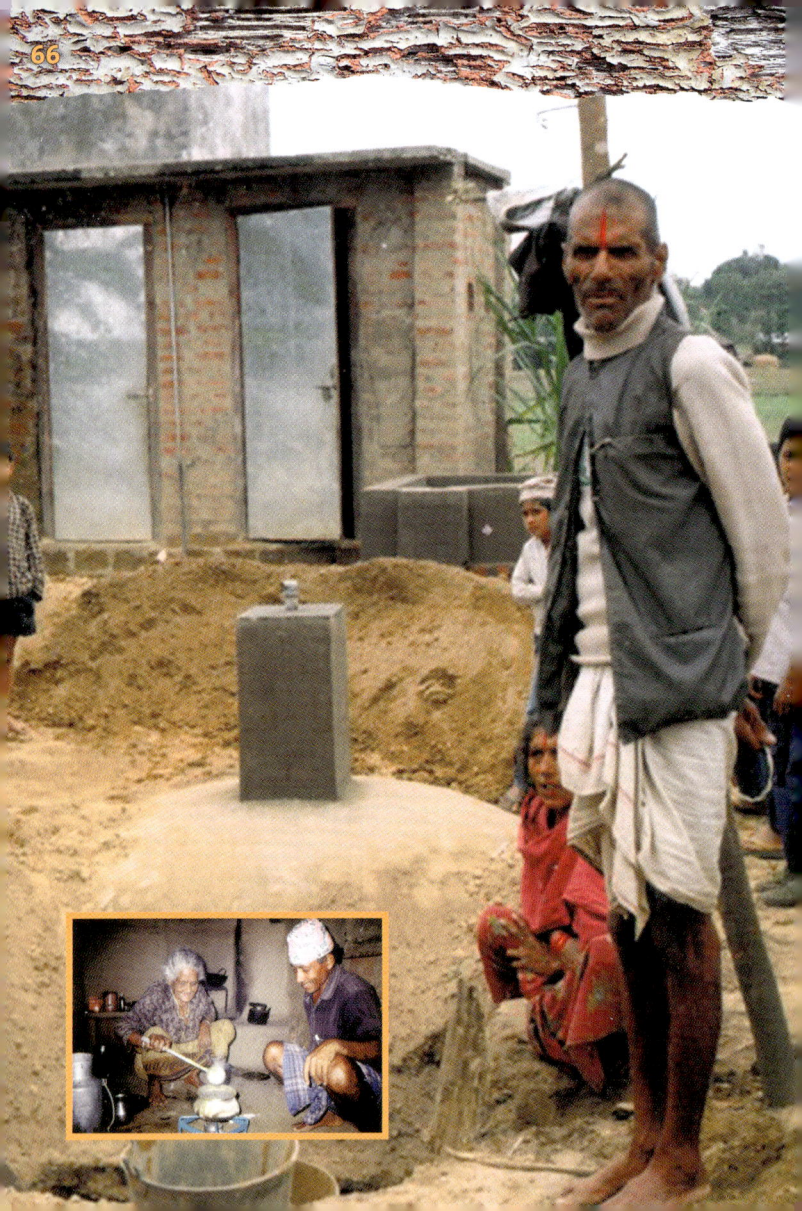

Some terminology used in this booklet

Black water	Water that contains excreta either from humans and/or from animals.
Excreta	Human waste: faeces and urine.
Faeces	Human waste matter discharged from the bowels.
Grey water	Household wastewater without any input of human and /or animal excreta.
Pathogen	An organism that creates diseases in a host.
Sewage	The spent or used water from a community that contains dissolved or suspended matter.
Sewerage	A drainage system involving sewers or pipes.
Urine	A pale-yellow fluid secreted as waste from the blood by the kidney and discharged through the urethra.
Wastewater	All types of domestic wastewater (sewage, grey water), commercial and industrial effluent as well as storm water runoff.

◁ Pour flush toilets connected with a biogas plant in Nepal
(photo SNV Netherlands Development Organisation).
Insert: Biogas used for cooking a meal in Nepal
(photo SNV Netherlands Development Organisation).

Call for information

Worldwide there are many examples of affordable, innovative and successful sanitation technologies which help to improve people's daily lives. Other people and communities can learn from these successes. This booklet presents you, the reader, an extensive selection of the 'state of the art' of existing affordable and sustainable sanitation options in their basic form. They offer a solution to the millions of households that do not yet have a proper sanitation facility nearby.

However, information about 'best practices' has to be accurate, up-to-date and easily accessible. It has to be easy to obtain, easy to understand and objective if it is to be useful to stakeholders.

Knowing the 'state of the art' about existing sanitation options is crucial for policymakers, financers, programme implementers, and is equally important for local industry and businesses looking for new products. All of these stakeholders need concise information about sanitation options, in order to make good decisions. The striving for sewered sanitation options has caused decision makers more or less to forget, or at least underestimate, the value of some of the non-sewered options. This booklet tries to fill this gap.

Some of the options described in this booklet are not new. Other technologies have recently been developed or are still under development. All are however technologies for practical action! In addition to giving examples, this booklet indicates that a great deal of flexibility is possible in combining different elements into a complete system. The booklet also refers to many other information sources and websites.

Organisations like IRC, WEDC, GTZ, EcoSanRes, WASTE, WSP and WHO disseminate information about smart technologies. They, along with other organisations mentioned in this booklet and in the third edition of Smart Water Solutions, will continue to update you about new smart technologies. However, there are probably other options, unknown to the authors, that also deserve a wider audience.

If you have experience of one or more such options, we invite you to share them with colleagues around the world. Please contact the NWP – www.nwp.nl